W9-AFR-394

Tobacco Information for Teens

Second Edition

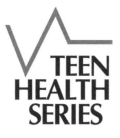

TEEN HEALTH SERIES

Second Edition

Tobacco Information for Teens

Health Tips about the Hazards of Using Cigarettes, Smokeless Tobacco, and Other Nicotine Products

Including Facts about Nicotine Addiction, Nicotine Delivery Systems, Secondhand Smoke, Health Consequences of Tobacco Use, Related Cancers, Smoking Cessation, and Tobacco Use Statistics

Edited by Karen Bellenir

P.O. Box 31-1640, Detroit, MI 48231

Bibliographic Note

Because this page cannot legibly accommodate all the copyright notices, the Bibliographic Note portion of the Preface constitutes an extension of the copyright notice.

Edited by Karen Bellenir

Teen Health Series

Karen Bellenir, *Managing Editor*
David A. Cooke, MD, FACP, *Medical Consultant*
Elizabeth Collins, *Research and Permissions Coordinator*
Cherry Edwards, *Permissions Assistant*
EdIndex, Services for Publishers, *Indexers*

* * *

Omnigraphics, Inc.

Matthew P. Barbour, *Senior Vice President*
Kevin M. Hayes, *Operations Manager*

* * *

Peter E. Ruffner, *Publisher*

Copyright © 2010 Omnigraphics, Inc.
ISBN 978-0-7808-1153-9

Library of Congress Cataloging-in-Publication Data

   Tobacco information for teens : health tips about the hazards of using cigarettes, smokeless tobacco, and other nicotine products : including facts about nicotine addiction, nicotine delivery systems, secondhand smoke, health consequences of tobacco use, related cancers, smoking cessation, and tobacco use statistics / edited by Karen Bellenir. -- 2nd ed.
      p. cm. -- (Teen health series)
   Includes bibliographical references and index.
      ISBN 978-0-7808-1153-9 (hardcover : alk. paper) 1. Tobacco use--Health aspects. 2. Smoking--Health aspects. 3. Nicotine--Health aspects. 4. Smoking cessation. 5. Teenagers--Tobacco use--Prevention. I. Bellenir, Karen.
   RA1242.T6T615 2010
   613.850835--dc22

                                                                                2010023716

∞

Table of Contents

Part Two: Nicotine Delivery Systems

Part Three: Cancers Associated With Tobacco Use

Part Four: Other Health Concerns Related To Tobacco Use

Part Five: Tobacco Use Cessation

Part Six: If You Need More Help Or Information

Preface

About This Book

Although most teens don't smoke—only 20% of high school students reported current cigarette use according to a recent report by the Centers for Disease Control and Prevention—national statistics indicate that every day approximately 4,000 U.S. adolescents between the ages of 12 and 17 try their first cigarette. The health consequences can be devastating. Cigarette smoking by young people leads to immediate and serious health problems, including respiratory and cardiovascular effects, changes in brain chemistry, and risks for nicotine addiction. Long-term smoking is linked to a host of life-threatening disorders, including various cancers, lung diseases, and heart attacks. In fact, an estimated one out of every five deaths in the United States is linked to cigarette smoking.

Tobacco Information for Teens, Second Edition offers updated information about the health consequences associated with smoking and other forms of tobacco use. It explains some of the cultural influences that can make tobacco use seem attractive and how teen curiosity can lead to nicotine-related problems. The various methods by which nicotine is consumed, including different types of cigarettes, cigars, hookah pipes, smokeless products, and even secondhand smoke, are explained. A section on cancers associated with tobacco describes the organs most commonly affected. A section on other health concerns related to tobacco use discusses some of the most common smoking-related diseases, including those that impact the heart, lungs, circulatory system, eyes, and sex organs. For teens who want to stop smoking—or help a friend or family member quit—facts about smoking cessation are included along with tips for dealing with the effects of nicotine withdrawal. The book concludes with directories of resources for more information.

How To Use This Book

This book is divided into parts and chapters. Parts focus on broad areas of interest; chapters are devoted to single topics within a part.

Part One: Facts About Tobacco And Nicotine provides data about the use of tobacco and other nicotine products. It explains how nicotine use leads to addiction, and it offers statistical information about the use of nicotine products in the United States and around the world. It also discusses legislative action concerning the sale and marketing of tobacco products.

Part Two: Nicotine Delivery Systems offers facts about the most common ways people consume or are exposed to nicotine. These include smoking different kinds of cigarettes, cigars, and pipes, using smokeless tobacco, and breathing secondhand smoke.

Part Three: Cancers Associated With Tobacco Use provides basic information about the types of cancer for which risks are most commonly linked to tobacco use. Although lung cancer is perhaps the most widely recognized cancer-related risk, others include bladder cancer, esophageal cancer, laryngeal cancer, oral cancer, and pancreatic cancer.

Part Four: Other Health Concerns Related To Tobacco Use explains how smoking and other tobacco use can lead to disease processes other than cancer that also harm the body's organs and systems. It discusses tobacco-related damage to the lungs, heart, blood vessels, and eyes, as well as adverse affects on sexual health and pregnancy outcomes.

Part Five: Tobacco Use Cessation offers information about quitting smoking or other types of tobacco use. It explains the use of nicotine replacement therapies, discusses medications commonly prescribed to aid in cessation efforts, and offers tips for coping with the effects of nicotine withdrawal.

Part Six: If You Need More Help Or Information provides directories of resources for obtaining more information about the health effects of tobacco use and smoking cessation.

Bibliographic Note

This volume contains documents and excerpts from publications issued by the following government agencies: Centers for Disease Control and Prevention; National Cancer Institute; National Center for Chronic Disease Prevention and Health Promotion; National Eye Institute; National Heart Lung and Blood Institute; National Institute of Dental and Craniofacial Research; National Institute of Diabetes and Digestive and Kidney Diseases; National Institute of Neurological Disorders and Stroke; National Institute on Drug Abuse; National Women's Health Information Center; Office of the Surgeon General; Substance Abuse and Mental Health Services Administration; U.S. Department of Defense; U.S. Environmental Protection Agency; and the U.S. Food and Drug Administration.

In addition, this volume contains copyrighted documents and articles produced by the following organizations: A.D.A.M., Inc.; American Academy of Orthopaedic Surgeons; American College of Chest Physicians; American Council on Science and Health; American Dental Hygienists' Association; American Legacy Foundation; BACCHUS Network; Campaign for Tobacco-Free Kids; March of Dimes Birth Defects Foundation; Nemours Foundation; New York State Smokers' Quitline; Ohio State University Medical Center; Planned Parenthood Federation of America, Inc.; Rhode Island Department of Health; Tobacco Control Legal Consortium; Tri-County Cessation Center; Trustees of Columbia University; and The World Bank.

The photograph on the front cover is from Pedro Tavares/Shutterstock Images LLC.

Full citation information is provided on the first page of each chapter. Every effort has been made to secure all necessary rights to reprint the copyrighted material. If any omissions have been made, please contact Omnigraphics to make corrections for future editions.

Acknowledgements

In addition to the organizations listed above, special thanks are due to Liz Collins, research and permissions coordinator; Cherry Edwards, permissions assistant; Zachary Klimecki, editorial assistant; and Elizabeth Bellenir, prepress technician.

About the *Teen Health Series*

At the request of librarians serving today's young adults, the *Teen Health Series* was developed as a specially focused set of volumes within Omnigraphics' *Health Reference Series*. Each volume deals comprehensively with a topic selected according to the needs and interests of people in middle school and high school.

Teens seeking preventive guidance, information about disease warning signs, medical statistics, and risk factors for health problems will find answers to their questions in the *Teen Health Series*. The *Series*, however, is not intended to serve as a tool for diagnosing illness, in prescribing treatments, or as a substitute for the physician/patient relationship. All people concerned about medical symptoms or the possibility of disease are encouraged to seek professional care from an appropriate health care provider.

If there is a topic you would like to see addressed in a future volume of the *Teen Health Series*, please write to:

Editor
Teen Health Series
Omnigraphics, Inc.
P.O. Box 31-1640
Detroit, MI 48231

A Note about Spelling and Style

Teen Health Series editors use *Stedman's Medical Dictionary* as an authority for questions related to the spelling of medical terms and the *Chicago Manual of Style* for questions related to grammatical structures, punctuation, and other editorial concerns. Consistent adherence is not always possible, however, because the individual volumes within the *Series* include many documents from a wide variety of different producers and copyright holders, and the editor's primary goal is to present material from each source as accurately as is possible following the terms specified by each document's producer. This sometimes means that information in different chapters or sections may follow other guidelines and alternate spelling authorities. For example, occasionally a copyright holder may require that eponymous terms be shown in possessive forms (Crohn's disease *vs.* Crohn disease) or that British spelling norms be retained (leukaemia *vs.* leukemia).

Locating Information within the *Teen Health Series*

The *Teen Health Series* contains a wealth of information about a wide variety of medical topics. As the *Series* continues to grow in size and scope, locating the precise information needed by a specific student may become more challenging. To address this concern, information about books within the *Teen Health Series* is included in *A Contents Guide to the Health Reference Series*. The *Contents Guide* presents an extensive list of more than 15,000 diseases, treatments, and other topics of general interest compiled from the Tables of Contents and major index headings from the books of the *Teen Health Series* and *Health Reference Series*. To access *A Contents Guide to the Health Reference Series*, visit www.healthreferenceseries.com.

Our Advisory Board

We would like to thank the following advisory board members for providing guidance to the development of this *Series*:

Dr. Lynda Baker, Associate Professor of Library and Information Science, Wayne State University, Detroit, MI

Nancy Bulgarelli, William Beaumont Hospital Library, Royal Oak, MI

Karen Imarisio, Bloomfield Township Public Library, Bloomfield Township, MI

Karen Morgan, Mardigian Library, University of Michigan-Dearborn, Dearborn, MI

Rosemary Orlando, St. Clair Shores Public Library, St. Clair Shores, MI

Medical Consultant

Medical consultation services are provided to the *Teen Health Series* editors by David A. Cooke, MD, FACP. Dr. Cooke is a graduate of Brandeis

University, and he received his M.D. degree from the University of Michigan. He completed residency training at the University of Wisconsin Hospital and Clinics. He is board-certified in internal medicine. Dr. Cooke currently works as part of the University of Michigan Health System and practices in Ann Arbor, MI. In his free time, he enjoys writing, science fiction, and spending time with his family.

Part One

Facts About Tobacco And Nicotine

Chapter 1

Smoking Stinks

Smoking is one of the worst things kids or adults can do to their bodies. Yet every single day about 4,000 kids between the ages 12 and 17 start smoking. Most middle school students don't smoke—only about one in 10 does. And most high school students don't smoke either—about one in four does (that means three out of four don't).

But why do those who smoke ever begin?

There's more than just one simple answer. Some kids may start smoking just because they're curious. Others may like the idea of doing something dangerous—something grownups don't want them to do. Still others might know lots of people who smoke and they might think it's a way to act or look like an adult. Fortunately, fewer people are starting smoking than a few years ago.

Maybe that's because more and more people have learned that smoking and tobacco use can cause cancer and heart disease. But sometimes kids can't really think that far into the future to worry about an illness they might not get for many years.

About This Chapter: Text in this chapter is from "Smoking Stinks," August 2007, reprinted with permission from www.kidshealth.org. Copyright © 2007 The Nemours Foundation. This information was provided by KidsHealth, one of the largest resources online for medically reviewed health information written for parents, kids, and teens. For more articles like this one, visit www.KidsHealth.org, or www.TeensHealth.org.

So let's talk about the problems that might affect kids more quickly:

- bad breath

- yellow teeth

- smelly clothes

- more colds and coughs

- difficulty keeping up with friends when playing sports

- empty wallet—cigarettes and tobacco products are very expensive

Let's find out more about cigarettes and tobacco.

> ✤ **It's A Fact!!**
>
> You won't see cigarettes advertised on TV or billboards, but cigarette companies still spend billions of dollars each year to promote their products. Have you ever seen an ad for cigarettes or tobacco? Did it make you want to try it?

What are smoking and smokeless tobacco?

Tobacco (say: tuh-ba-ko) is a plant that can be smoked in cigarettes, pipes, or cigars. It's the same plant that's in smokeless tobacco, known as dip, chew, snuff, spit, or chewing tobacco. Smokeless tobacco is not lit or inhaled like tobacco in cigarettes, pipes, and cigars. Instead, smokeless tobacco is put between the lip and gum and sucked on inside the mouth.

Tobacco contains nicotine (say: nih-kuh-teen), a chemical that causes a tingly or pleasant feeling—but that feeling only lasts for a little while. Nicotine is also addictive (say: uh-dik-tiv). That means that if you start to use nicotine, your body and mind will become so used to it that you'll need to have it just to feel OK.

Anyone who starts smoking could become addicted to it. If you're addicted to something, it's very hard to stop doing it, even if you want to. Some kids get addicted right away. And adults are often addicted, which is why so many of them have a hard time quitting smoking.

Why is it so bad for you?

Cigarettes and smokeless tobacco kill hundreds of thousands of Americans every year. You know those rubber bracelets that were created to bring attention to different causes? The Campaign for Tobacco-Free Kids created a red one with the number 1,200 on it. Why 1,200? That's the number of people who die each day due to smoking.

The nicotine and other poisonous chemicals in tobacco cause lots of diseases, like heart problems and some kinds of cancer. If you smoke, you hurt your lungs and heart each time you light up. It also can make it more difficult for blood to move around in the body, so smokers may feel tired and cranky. The longer you smoke, the worse the damage becomes.

What's it like?

Usually, people don't like smoking or chewing tobacco at first. Your body is smart, and it knows when it's being poisoned. When people try smoking for the first time, they often cough a lot and feel pain or burning in their throat and lungs. This is your lungs' way of trying to protect you and tell you to keep them smoke free. Also, many people say that they feel sick to their stomachs or even throw up. If someone accidentally swallows chewing tobacco, they may be sick for hours. Yuck.

What if my friend smokes?

If you have friends who smoke or use tobacco, you can help them by encouraging them to quit. Here are some reasons you can mention:

- It will hurt their health.

- It will make their breath stinky.

- It will turn their teeth yellow.

✤ It's A Fact!!
The Other Cost Of Smoking

Using tobacco eats up a lot of money, too. A pack of cigarettes costs $4.50, on average. That means, even if you buy just one pack a week, you'll spend $234 in a year. Some people smoke a pack a day, which adds up to $1,642. That's a lot of CDs, computer games, and clothes you could buy instead.

- It will give them less endurance when running or playing sports.

- It's expensive.

- It's illegal to buy cigarettes when you're underage.

If you think it will help, you could print out articles like this one to give to a friend who smokes. He or she may be interested in learning more about the dangers of smoking. But people don't like to hear that they're doing something wrong, so your pal also could be a little angry. If that happens, don't push it too much. In time, your friend may realize you are right.

In the meantime, it could help to talk with a parent or a school counselor if you're worried about your friend. When your friend is ready, a grown-up can help him or her quit for good. If your friend decides to quit, lend your support. You might say it's time to kick some butts.

Chapter 2

Debunking The Myths About Tobacco

Cigarette Smoking Is Bad For You

You knew that. Almost everybody knows that. After all, there have been warning labels on cigarette packages since before you were born.

But the problem with warning labels is that they're short—far too short to give you the complete picture of what cigarettes can do to your body. To give you all of the facts you need about cigarette smoking, it would be necessary to have a warning label the size of a book.

The people at the American Council on Science and Health created this information because we want you to have the facts—all of the facts—about smoking. We designed this information especially for people your age because knowing the truth about smoking is particularly important for you.

You see, most smokers start to smoke while they are in middle school or high school. Almost 90% of all smokers start to smoke before reaching the age of 18. People make the decision to smoke—one of the most important decisions of their lives—when they are your age or just a little bit older. And unfortunately, many of them don't have all the facts about cigarettes when they decide to start smoking. In fact, some of them believe myths about smoking that are just plain wrong.

About This Chapter: Excerpted from "The Scoop On Smoking from ACSH," © 2009 American Council on Science and Health. Reprinted with permission. For additional information, visit http://thescooponsmoking.org.

So let's start by talking about ten common myths about smoking—none of which is mentioned on the warning labels.

Myths Debunked

Myth #1: Most people smoke.

Actually, most people don't smoke. This is true both for adults and for teenagers.

- Among adults in the U.S., 77% are nonsmokers.

- Among high school students, 71% are nonsmokers.

If all of these people don't smoke, you don't have to either.

Myth #2: Smoking is cool.

Actually, most teenagers don't think that smoking is cool. In fact,

- 67% of teenagers say that seeing someone smoke turns them off.

- 65% say that they strongly dislike being around smokers.

- 86% would rather date people who don't smoke.

Many teenagers think that kissing a smoker is like licking a dirty ashtray; perhaps this is why the percentage who don't want to date smokers is so high.

If you've gotten the impression that smoking is cool, it may be because smoking is portrayed that way in cigarette advertising. Ads for cigarettes—like ads for other products—are designed to associate the product with positive images. Cigarette ads usually show smiling, healthy-looking young adults, in an outdoor setting, having fun with friends. That's a "cool" image. But letting advertising manipulate you into making poor choices is not cool. What's really cool is thinking for yourself and making smart personal decisions.

♣ It's A Fact!!

Even teenagers who smoke don't think that smoking is cool. More than half of all teenage smokers want to quit, and about 70% of teenage smokers wish that they had never started smoking in the first place.

Myth #3: Sure, smoking is unhealthy. But a lot of other things are just as bad for you. After all, practically everything seems to have a warning label.

Smoking is far, far worse than most other health hazards. Let's look at some of the numbers:

- Smoking is the number one cause of avoidable deaths in the United States.

- Every year, more than 400,000 Americans die as a result of smoking.

- One out of every five deaths in the U.S. is due to smoking.

- Worldwide, four million people a year die from smoking—that's 11,000 people every day.

- Smoking kills one-half of all people who smoke.

To put the impact of smoking into perspective, it may help to consider six other major causes of death in the United States: alcohol abuse, drug abuse, AIDS, motor vehicle crashes, homicide, and suicide. All of these are important problems. All of them kill substantial numbers of people every year. Yet all six of these causes combined account for only half as many deaths each year as smoking does.

Let's try another comparison. For the rest of your life, you will undoubtedly remember the terrorist attacks on the World Trade Center and the Pentagon that occurred on September 11, 2001. About 3,000 people died in those attacks. But that number is small compared to the number of people killed by smoking every year. In fact, cigarette smoking kills that many Americans every three days.

Of course, cigarettes aren't the only products that carry warning labels. If you look around your home, you can probably find warning labels on a lot of other products. For example:

- Your hair dryer has a warning label that tells you that you shouldn't use it while taking a bath because you could be electrocuted.

- The plastic bags that you bring home from the grocery store have warning labels saying that they can suffocate small children.

- The charcoal that your parents use in their barbecue grill has a warning label that says that it shouldn't be used indoors because it could cause carbon monoxide poisoning.

How do the hazards of these products compare to the hazards of cigarettes?

- Each year, an average of four Americans are electrocuted by hair dryers.
- Each year, approximately 25 U.S. children are suffocated by plastic bags.
- Each year, roughly 20 Americans are killed by carbon monoxide poisoning due to the indoor burning of charcoal.
- Each year, more than 400,000 Americans are killed by cigarette smoking.

In other words, the other three products aren't even in the same league with cigarettes.

There's another important difference between the other three products and cigarettes. Hair dryers, plastic bags, and charcoal are all safe if you use them correctly. They're only dangerous if you misuse them.

Cigarettes are deadly when they're used in the way that they're supposed to be used. There is no such thing as a "safe" cigarette.

Cigarettes are harmful to everyone who uses them. This is different from the situation for some other products that carry warning labels. Let's consider a warning label that most people your age have seen many times—the warning on video games that tells you that light flashes in the games can cause some people to have seizures. How does this hazard compare to the hazard of smoking cigarettes?

- One out of every 4,000 people is at risk of having a seizure from light flashes associated with video games.
- 4,000 out of every 4,000 people are at risk of damaging their health by smoking cigarettes.

Please don't misunderstand us here. We're not saying that warning labels on products such as hair dryers and video games aren't justified. Those labels give people useful information, and they may help to save lives. It's a good idea to have them. But don't let the proliferation of warning labels fool you into thinking that cigarettes are "just like everything else." They're not. Cigarettes are worse. Much worse.

Myth #4: Smoking only causes a few health problems—the ones listed on the warning labels.

The only health problems specifically mentioned on the warning labels are lung cancer, heart disease, emphysema, and special problems that can happen when a pregnant woman smokes (complications of pregnancy, injury to the unborn child, low birth weight, and premature birth). But smoking also increases your risk of a wide variety of other diseases. And for people who already have health problems, smoking can make many of those problems worse.

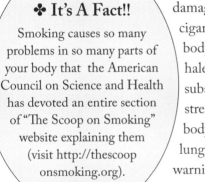

✦ It's A Fact!!

Smoking causes so many problems in so many parts of your body that the American Council on Science and Health has devoted an entire section of "The Scoop on Smoking" website explaining them (visit http://thescoop onsmoking.org).

Smoking is able to cause such widespread damage because harmful substances from cigarette smoke reach every part of your body. Within seconds after a person inhales cigarette smoke, about 4,000 toxic substances are absorbed into the bloodstream. They then travel to every cell in the body. Thus, smoking doesn't just affect your lungs and heart—it affects everything. But warning labels that mention only heart and lung diseases and pregnancy problems don't give people this message.

Myth #5: Smoking won't affect my health until I'm much older.

Actually, if you smoke now, it can hurt you now. Some of the harmful effects of smoking occur right away.

You also need to know that smoking-related diseases can kill people at surprisingly young ages. Some of the victims are in their thirties or forties. For example:

- Nancy Gore Hunger, sister of former Vice President Al Gore, died of lung cancer due to smoking at 46.

- Actress Carrie Hamilton, daughter of TV star Carol Burnett, died of lung cancer due to smoking at 38.

You were planning to live a lot longer than these people did, weren't you?

Myth #6: I only smoke a little. That won't hurt me.

Even smoking a little can hurt you. Research has shown that even "occasional" (less-than-daily) smoking, smoking only a few cigarettes per day, or smoking "without inhaling" can increase your risk of heart disease and shorten your life.

Actually, the idea that smoking "just a little" can be harmful to your health should not come as a surprise. The amount of tobacco smoke exposure that results from occasional smoking is similar to the amount that results from frequent exposure to tobacco smoke in the environment. Scientists know that exposure to environmental tobacco smoke can be harmful to your health. So it makes sense that smoking just a little would also be unhealthy.

In terms of health effects, cigarette smoking is quite different from eating candy or drinking coffee. People can consume candy and coffee in moderate amounts without hurting themselves. It's only when they go overboard and use these things to excess that they get into trouble. But there is no such thing as smoking "in moderation." Any amount of smoking is bad for you.

In terms of health effects, smoking is also very different from going out in the sun. You probably know that a little exposure to sunlight is good for you; it helps your body make vitamin D. But too much exposure to the sun can give you a sunburn and increase your chances of getting skin cancer. Smoking is not like this. There is no beneficial level of smoking. While it is true that smoking may actually protect against a few diseases such as Parkinson's (a disease of the nervous system), probably as a result of the actions of nicotine (a drug found in tobacco), these potential benefits are more than outweighed by the extensive harm caused by tobacco smoke's other effects in the body.

Another problem with smoking "just a little" is that most people can't do it for long. Cigarettes are physically addictive. If you become a smoker, your body will adapt to cigarettes so that you will come to need them—and need them several times a day—in order to feel normal. Because cigarettes are addictive, most people can't continue to be occasional smokers for long. Soon, they find themselves smoking every day, several times a day. And the more they smoke, the more they are damaging their health.

Myth #7: I'm only going to smoke for a few years. Then I'll quit. So my smoking doesn't really matter.

People who assume that all of the health hazards of cigarettes will disappear in a puff of smoke when they quit are wrong—dead wrong. Many of the harmful effects of smoking are irreversible, meaning that they do not go away completely after a person quits smoking.

Smoking for as short a time as five years can cause permanent damage—to the lungs, heart, eyes, throat, urinary tract, digestive organs, bones and joints, and skin. Although it is true, as one of the cigarette warning labels says, that quitting smoking reduces health risks, many of those risks are only partially reversible. Ex-smokers continue to have increased risks of many smoking-related diseases and health problems, including lung cancer, bladder cancer, chronic obstructive lung disease, the bone disease osteoporosis, serious diseases of the eyes (cataracts and macular degeneration), and muscle and bone pain. Only for heart disease and stroke is there good evidence that the risk faced by an ex-smoker ever returns to that of a lifelong nonsmoker—and even that takes from five to 15 years after a person quits smoking.

♣ It's A Fact!!

Scientists estimate that between 10 and 37% of ex-smokers will die from diseases caused by their smoking. Although this is certainly better than the situation among people who continue to smoke (about half of whom will die of smoking), it is a clear indicator that some of the harm caused by smoking cannot be undone.

In addition, for many people, smoking itself is irreversible. Even with multiple attempts and the help of modern quit-smoking techniques, many smokers never succeed in stopping smoking permanently. The addictive power of nicotine is so strong that millions of people continue to smoke even though they know that cigarettes may kill them.

Myth #8: Smoking will help me lose weight.

Actually, it won't. Starting to smoke is not associated with a decrease in body weight. Unfortunately, though, quitting smoking is followed by a gain in weight for many people.

So here's what's likely to happen if you start to smoke in the hope of losing weight:

- You start smoking.
- After a while, you realize that your weight has not changed. You're disappointed.
- Then you realize that instead of a better-looking body, what you have is a smelly, dirty, unattractive, expensive, dangerous addiction. You're horrified.
- You quit smoking. It's tough, but you manage to do it.
- You gain weight. Now you're heavier than you were when you started.

Does this make sense?

Myth #9: I don't smoke cigarettes. I just smoke cigars or bidis or use smokeless tobacco. So I don't have a problem.

Actually, you do have a problem. All of these other forms of tobacco are addictive, and all are seriously harmful to your health. You can find the facts about cigars, bidis, and smokeless tobacco on The Scoop on Smoking website (http://thescooponsmoking.org).

Myth #10: OK. I admit that smoking is bad for me. But that's my problem, not anybody else's. The only person I'm hurting is me, so it's nobody else's business.

Well, first of all, your smoking is a problem for all of the people who care about you. They don't like to see you harming yourself, and they would be thrilled if you would quit.

But beyond that, there's another problem. When you smoke, your cigarettes give off smoke into the environment. That smoke is harmful to other people's health. It's especially harmful to children—and that's important, because in another ten years or so, you may be starting a family. The last people in the world that you would want to hurt are your own children, but if you're a smoker, you may find yourself doing that. Women who smoke can even harm their children before they're born because smoking during pregnancy is bad for the baby.

So I guess it would be better if I never started smoking, right?

Exactly. But you may still want more information before you make such an important decision. In particular, you may want to know how smoking can affect your health right now. To find out, check out the effects section of this website: http://thescooponsmoking.org.

Chapter 3

Chemicals In Tobacco Smoke

The list of 599 additives approved by the U.S. Government for use in the manufacture of cigarettes is something every smoker should see. Submitted by the five major American cigarette companies to the Department of Health and Human Services in April of 1994, this list of ingredients had long been kept a secret.

Tobacco companies reporting this information were:

- American Tobacco Company

- Brown and Williamson

- Liggett Group, Inc.

- Philip Morris Inc.

- R.J. Reynolds Tobacco Company

While these ingredients are approved as additives for foods, they were not tested by burning them, and it is the burning of many of these substances which changes their properties, often for the worse. Over 4000 chemical compounds are created by burning a cigarette. Sixty-nine of those chemicals are known to cause cancer. Carbon monoxide, nitrogen oxides, hydrogen cyanides and ammonia are all present in cigarette smoke. Forty-three known carcinogens are

About This Chapter: Text in this chapter is from "Cigarette Ingredients," © Tri-County Cessation Center (www.tricountycessation.org). Reprinted with permission.

in mainstream smoke, sidestream smoke, or both. It's chilling to think about not only how smokers poison themselves, but what others are exposed to by breathing in the secondhand smoke. The next time you're missing your old buddy, the cigarette, take a good long look at this list and see them for what they are: a delivery system for toxic chemical and carcinogens.

More Ingredients In A Cigarette

- Acetanisole

- Acetic acid

- Acetoin

- Acetophenone

- 6-Acetoxydihydrotheaspirane

- 2-Acetyl-3- ethylpyrazine

- 2-Acetyl-5-methylfuran

- Acetylpyrazine

- 2-Acetylpyridine

- 3-Acetylpyridine

- 2-Acetylthiazole

- Aconitic acid

- dl-Alanine

- Alfalfa extract

- Allspice extract, oleoresin, and oil

- Allyl hexanoate

- Allyl ionone

- Almond bitter oil

- Ambergris tincture

- Ammonia

- Ammonium bicarbonate

> ### ✤ It's A Fact!!
> There are over 4,000 chemicals in tobacco smoke and at least 69 of those chemicals are known to cause cancer.

- Ammonium hydroxide

- Ammonium phosphate dibasic

- Ammonium sulfide

- Amyl alcohol

- Amyl butyrate

- Amyl formate

- Amyl octanoate

- alpha-Amylcinnamaldehyde

- Amyris oil

- trans-anethole

- Angelica root extract, oil and seed oil

- Anise

- Anise star, extract and oils

- Anisyl acetate
- Anisyl alcohol
- Anisyl formate
- Anisyl phenylacetate
- Apple juice concentrate, extract, and skins
- Apricot extract and juice concentrate
- 1-Arginine
- Asafetida fluid extract and oil
- Ascorbic acid
- 1-Asparagine monohydrate
- 1-Aspartic acid
- Balsam Peru and oil
- Basil oil
- Bay leaf, oil and sweet oil
- Beeswax white
- Beet juice concentrate
- Benzaldehyde
- Benzaldehyde glyceryl acetal
- Benzoic acid, benzoin
- Benzoin resin
- Benzophenone
- Benzyl alcohol
- Benzyl benzoate
- Benzyl butyrate
- Benzyl cinnamate
- Benzyl propionate
- Benzyl salicylate
- Bergamot oil
- Bisabolene
- Black currant buds absolute
- Borneol
- Bornyl acetate
- Buchu leaf oil
- 1,3-Butanediol
- 2,3-Butanedione
- 1-Butanol
- 2-Butanone
- 4(2-Butenylidene)-3,5,5-trimethyl-2-cyclohexen-1-one
- Butter, butter esters, and butter oil
- Butyl acetate
- Butyl butyrate
- Butyl butyryl lactate
- Butyl isovalerate
- Butyl phenylacetate
- Butyl undecylenate
- 3-Butylidenephthalide
- Butyric acid
- Cadinene
- Caffeine
- Calcium carbonate

- Camphene
- Cananga oil
- Capsicum oleoresin
- Caramel color
- Caraway oil
- Carbon dioxide
- Cardamom oleoresin, extract, seed oil, and powder
- Carob bean and extract
- beta-Carotene
- Carrot oil
- Carvacrol
- 4-Carvomenthenol
- 1-Carvone
- beta-Caryophyllene
- beta-Caryophyllene oxide
- Cascarilla oil and bark extract
- Cassia bark oil
- Cassie absolute and oil
- Castoreum extract, tincture and absolute
- Cedar leaf oil
- Cedarwood oil terpenes and virginiana
- Cedrol
- Celery seed extract, solid, oil, and oleoresin
- Cellulose fiber
- Chamomile flower oil and extract
- Chicory extract
- Chocolate
- Cinnamaldehyde
- Cinnamic acid
- Cinnamon leaf oil, bark oil, and extract
- Cinnamyl acetate
- Cinnamyl alcohol
- Cinnamyl cinnamate
- Cinnamyl isovalerate
- Cinnamyl propionate
- Citral
- Citric acid
- Citronella oil
- dl-Citronellol
- Citronellyl butyrate
- Citronellyl isobutyrate
- Civet absolute
- Clary oil
- Clover tops, red solid extract
- Cocoa
- Cocoa shells, extract, distillate and powder
- Coconut oil
- Coffee
- Cognac white and green oil

- Copaiba oil
- Coriander extract and oil
- Corn oil
- Corn silk
- Costus root oil
- Cubeb oil
- Cuminaldehyde
- para-Cymene
- 1-Cysteine dandelion root solid extract
- Davana oil
- 2-trans, 4-trans-Decadienal
- delta-Decalactone
- gamma-Decalactone
- Decanal
- Decanoic acid
- 1-Decanol
- 2-Decenal
- Dehydromenthofurolactone
- Diethyl malonate
- Diethyl sebacate
- 2,3-Diethylpyrazine
- Dihydro anethole
- 5,7-Dihydro-2-methylthieno(3,4-D) pyrimidine
- Dill seed oil and extract
- meta-Dimethoxybenzene
- para-Dimethoxybenzene
- 2,6-Dimethoxyphenol
- Dimethyl succinate
- 3,4-Dimethyl-1,2 cyclopentanedione
- 3,5- Dimethyl-1,2-cyclopentanedione
- 3,7-Dimethyl-1,3,6-octatriene
- 4,5-Dimethyl-3-hydroxy-2,5-dihydrofuran-2-one
- 6,10-Dimethyl-5,9-undecadien-2-one
- 3,7-Dimethyl-6-octenoic acid
- 2,4 Dimethylacetophenone
- alpha,para-Dimethylbenzyl alcohol
- alpha,alpha-Dimethylphenethyl acetate
- alpha,alpha Dimethylphenethyl butyrate
- 2,3-Dimethylpyrazine
- 2,5-Dimethylpyrazine
- 2,6-Dimethylpyrazine
- Dimethyltetrahydrobenzofuranone
- delta-Dodecalactone
- gamma-Dodecalactone
- para-Ethoxybenzaldehyde
- Ethyl 10-undecenoate
- Ethyl 2-methylbutyrate
- Ethyl acetate

- Ethyl acetoacetate
- Ethyl alcohol
- Ethyl benzoate
- Ethyl butyrate
- Ethyl cinnamate
- Ethyl decanoate
- Ethyl fenchol
- Ethyl furoate
- Ethyl heptanoate
- Ethyl hexanoate
- Ethyl isovalerate
- Ethyl lactate
- Ethyl laurate
- Ethyl levulinate
- Ethyl maltol
- Ethyl methyl phenylglycidate
- Ethyl myristate
- Ethyl nonanoate
- Ethyl octadecanoate
- Ethyl octanoate
- Ethyl oleate
- Ethyl palmitate
- Ethyl phenylacetate
- Ethyl propionate
- Ethyl salicylate
- Ethyl trans-2-butenoate
- Ethyl valerate
- Ethyl vanillin
- 2-Ethyl (or methyl)-(3,5 and 6)-methoxypyrazine
- 2-Ethyl-1-hexanol, 3-ethyl -2 - hydroxy-2-cyclopenten-1-one
- 2-Ethyl-3, (5 or 6)-dimethyl-pyrazine
- 5-Ethyl-3-hydroxy-4-methyl-2 (5H)-furanone
- 2-Ethyl-3-methylpyrazine
- 4-Ethylbenzaldehyde
- 4-Ethylguaiacol
- para-Ethylphenol
- 3-Ethylpyridine
- Eucalyptol
- Farnesol
- d-Fenchone
- Fennel sweet oil
- Fenugreek, extract, resin, and absolute
- Fig juice concentrate
- Food starch modified
- Furfuryl mercaptan
- 4-(2-Furyl)-3-buten-2-one
- Galbanum oil
- Genet absolute
- Gentian root extract
- Geraniol
- Geranium rose oil
- Geranyl acetate

- Geranyl butyrate
- Geranyl formate
- Geranyl isovalerate
- Geranyl phenylacetate
- Ginger oil and oleoresin
- 1-Glutamic acid
- 1-Glutamine
- Glycerol
- Glycyrrhizin ammoniated
- Grape juice concentrate
- Guaiac wood oil
- Guaiacol
- Guar gum
- 2,4-Heptadienal
- gamma-Heptalactone
- Heptanoic acid
- 2-Heptanone
- 3-Hepten-2-one
- 2-Hepten-4-one
- 4-Heptenal
- trans -2-Heptenal
- Heptyl acetate
- omega-6-Hexadecenlactone
- gamma-Hexalactone
- Hexanal
- Hexanoic acid
- 2-Hexen-1-ol
- 3-Hexen-1-ol
- cis-3-Hexen-1-yl acetate
- 2-Hexenal
- 3-Hexenoic acid
- trans-2-Hexenoic acid
- cis-3-Hexenyl formate
- Hexyl 2-methylbutyrate
- Hexyl acetate
- Hexyl alcohol
- Hexyl phenylacetate
- 1-Histidine
- Honey
- Hops oil
- Hydrolyzed milk solids
- Hydrolyzed plant proteins
- 5-Hydroxy-2,4-decadienoic acid delta-lactone
- 4-Hydroxy-2,5-dimethyl-3(2H)-furanone
- 2-Hydroxy-3,5,5-trimethyl-2-cyclohexen-1-one
- 4-Hydroxy-3-pentenoic acid lactone
- 2-Hydroxy-4-methylbenzalde-hyde
- 4-Hydroxybutanoic acid lac-tone
- Hydroxycitronellal
- 6-Hydroxydihydrotheaspirane
- 4-(para-Hydroxyphenyl)-2-butanone

- Hyssop oil
- Immortelle absolute and extract
- alpha-Ionone
- beta-Ionone
- alpha-Irone
- Isoamyl acetate
- Isoamyl benzoate
- Isoamyl butyrate
- Isoamyl cinnamate
- Isoamyl formate, isoamyl-hexanoate
- Isoamyl isovalerate
- Isoamyl octanoate
- Isoamyl phenylacetate
- Isobornyl acetate
- Isobutyl acetate
- Isobutyl alcohol
- Isobutyl cinnamate
- Isobutyl phenylacetate
- Isobutyl salicylate
- 2-Isobutyl-3-methoxypyrazine
- Alpha-isobutylphenethyl alcohol
- Isobutyraldehyde
- Isobutyric acid
- d,l-Isoleucine
- alpha-Isomethylionone
- 2-Isopropylphenol
- Isovaleric acid
- Jasmine absolute, concrete and oil
- Kola nut extract
- Labdanum absolute and oleoresin
- Lactic acid
- Lauric acid
- Lauric aldehyde
- Lavandin oil
- Lavender oil
- Lemon oil and extract
- Lemongrass oil
- 1-Leucine
- Levulinic acid
- Licorice root, fluid, extract and powder
- Lime oil
- Linalool
- Linalool oxide
- Linalyl acetate
- Linden flowers
- Lovage oil and extract
- 1-Lysine
- Mace powder, extract and oil
- Magnesium carbonate
- Malic acid
- Malt and malt extract

- Maltodextrin
- Maltol
- Maltyl isobutyrate
- Mandarin oil
- Maple syrup and concentrate
- Mate leaf, absolute and oil
- para-Mentha-8-thiol-3-one
- Menthol
- Menthone
- Menthyl acetate
- dl-Methionine
- Methoprene
- 2-Methoxy-4-methylphenol
- 2-Methoxy-4-vinylphenol
- para-Methoxybenzaldehyde
- 1-(para-Methoxyphenyl)-1-penten-3-one
- 4-(para-Methoxyphenyl)-2-butanone
- 1-(para-Methoxyphenyl)-2-propanone
- Methoxypyrazine
- Methyl 2-furoate
- Methyl 2-octynoate
- Methyl 2-pyrrolyl ketone
- Methyl anisate
- Methyl anthranilate
- Methyl benzoate
- Methyl cinnamate
- Methyl dihydrojasmonate
- Methyl ester of rosin, partially hydrogenated
- Methyl isovalerate
- Methyl linoleate (48%)
- Methyl linolenate (52%) mixture
- Methyl naphthyl ketone
- Methyl nicotinate
- Methyl phenylacetate
- Methyl salicylate
- Methyl sulfide
- 3-Methyl-1-cyclopentadecanone
- 4-Methyl-1-phenyl-2-pentanone
- 5-Methyl-2-phenyl-2-hexenal
- 5-Methyl-2-thiophene-carboxaldehyde
- 6-Methyl-3,-5-heptadien-2-one
- 2-Methyl-3-(para-isopropyl-phenyl) propionaldehyde
- 5-Methyl-3-hexen-2-one
- 1-Methyl-3methoxy-4-isopropylbenzene
- 4-Methyl-3-pentene-2-one
- 2-Methyl-4-phenylbutyraldehyde

- 6-Methyl-5-hepten-2-one
- 4-Methyl-5-thiazoleethanol
- 4-Methyl-5-vinylthiazole
- Methyl-alpha-ionone
- Methyl-trans-2-butenoic acid
- 4-Methylacetophenone
- para-Methylanisole
- alpha-Methylbenzyl acetate
- alpha-Methylbenzyl alcohol
- 2-Methylbutyraldehyde
- 3-Methylbutyraldehyde
- 2-Methylbutyric acid
- alpha-Methylcinnamaldehyde
- Methylcyclopentenolone
- 2-Methylheptanoic acid
- 2-Methylhexanoic acid
- 3-Methylpentanoic acid
- 4-Methylpentanoic acid
- 2-Methylpyrazine
- 5-Methylquinoxaline
- 2-Methyltetrahydrofuran-3-one
- (Methylthio)methylpyrazine (mixture of isomers)
- 3-Methylthiopropionaldehyde
- Methyl 3-methylthiopropionate
- 2-Methylvaleric acid
- Mimosa absolute and extract
- Molasses extract and tincture
- Mountain maple solid extract
- Mullein flowers
- Myristaldehyde
- Myristic acid
- Myrrh oil
- beta-Napthyl ethyl ether
- Nerol
- Neroli bigarde oil
- Nerolidol
- Nona-2-trans,6-cis-dienal
- 2,6-Nonadien-1-ol
- gamma-Nonalactone
- Nonanal
- Nonanoic acid
- Nonanone
- trans-2-Nonen-1-ol
- 2-Nonenal
- Nonyl acetate
- Nutmeg powder and oil
- Oak chips extract and oil
- Oak moss absolute
- 9,12-Octadecadienoic acid (48%) and 9,12,15-octadeca-trienoic acid (52%)
- delta-Octalactone
- gamma-Octalactone
- Octanal
- Octanoic acid
- 1-Octanol

- 2-Octanone
- 3-Octen-2-one
- 1-Octen-3-ol
- 1-Octen-3-yl acetate
- 2-Octenal
- Octyl isobutyrate
- Oleic acid
- Olibanum oil
- Opoponax oil and gum
- Orange blossoms water, absolute, and leaf absolute
- Orange oil and extract
- Origanum oil
- Orris concrete oil and root extract
- Palmarosa oil
- Palmitic acid
- Parsley seed oil
- Patchouli oil
- omega-Pentadecalactone
- 2,3-Pentanedione
- 2-Pentanone
- 4-Pentenoic acid
- 2-Pentylpyridine
- Pepper oil, black and white
- Peppermint oil
- Peruvian (bois de rose) oil
- Petitgrain absolute, mandarin oil and terpeneless oil
- alpha-Phellandrene
- 2-Phenenthyl acetate
- Phenenthyl alcohol
- Phenethyl butyrate
- Phenethyl cinnamate
- Phenethyl isobutyrate
- Phenethyl isovalerate
- Phenethyl phenylacetate
- Phenethyl salicylate
- 1-Phenyl-1-propanol
- 3-Phenyl-1-propanol
- 2-Phenyl-2-butenal
- 4-Phenyl-3-buten-2-ol
- 4-Phenyl-3-buten-2-one
- Phenylacetaldehyde
- Phenylacetic acid
- 1-Phenylalanine
- 3-Phenylpropionaldehyde
- 3-Phenylpropionic acid
- 3-Phenylpropyl acetate
- 3-Phenylpropyl cinnamate
- 2-(3-Phenylpropyl)tetra-hydrofuran
- Phosphoric acid
- Pimenta leaf oil
- Pine needle oil, pine oil, scotch
- Pineapple juice concentrate
- alpha-Pinene, beta-pinene

- d-Piperitone
- Piperonal
- Pipsissewa leaf extract
- Plum juice
- Potassium sorbate
- 1-Proline
- Propenylguaethol
- Propionic acid
- Propyl acetate
- Propyl para-hydroxybenzoate
- Propylene glycol
- 3-Propylidenephthalide
- Prune juice and concentrate
- Pyridine
- Pyroligneous acid and extract
- Pyrrole
- Pyruvic acid
- Raisin juice concentrate
- Rhodinol
- Rose absolute and oil
- Rosemary oil
- Rum
- Rum ether
- Rye extract
- Sage, sage oil, and sage oleoresin
- Salicylaldehyde
- Sandalwood oil, yellow
- Sclareolide
- Skatole
- Smoke flavor
- Snakeroot oil
- Sodium acetate
- Sodium benzoate
- Sodium bicarbonate
- Sodium carbonate
- Sodium chloride
- Sodium citrate
- Sodium hydroxide
- Solanone
- Spearmint oil
- Styrax extract, gum and oil
- Sucrose octaacetate
- Sugar alcohols
- Sugars
- Tagetes oil
- Tannic acid
- Tartaric acid
- Tea leaf and absolute
- alpha-Terpineol
- Terpinolene
- Terpinyl acetate
- 5,6,7,8-Tetrahydroquinoxaline
- 1,5,5,9-Tetramethyl-13-oxatri-cyclo(8.3.0.0(4,9))tridecane
- 2,3,4,5, and 3,4,5,6-Tetra-methylethyl-cyclohexanone

- 2,3,5,6-Tetramethylpyrazine
- Thiamine hydrochloride
- Thiazole
- 1-Threonine
- Thyme oil, white and red
- Thymol
- Tobacco extracts
- Tochopherols (mixed)
- Tolu balsam gum and extract
- Tolualdehydes
- para-Tolyl 3-methylbutyrate
- para-Tolyl acetaldehyde
- para-Tolyl acetate
- para-Tolyl isobutyrate
- para-Tolyl phenylacetate
- Triacetin
- 2-Tridecanone
- 2-Tridecenal
- Triethyl citrate
- 3,5,5-Trimethyl -1-hexanol
- para,alpha,alpha-Trimethyl-benzyl alcohol
- 4-(2,6,6-Trimethylcyclohex-1-enyl)but-2-en-4-one
- 2,6,6-Trimethylcyclohex-2-ene-1,4-dione
- 2,6,6-Trimethylcyclohexa-1,3-dienyl methan
- 4-(2,6,6-Trimethylcyclohexa-1,3-dienyl)but-2-en-4-one
- 2,2,6-Trimethylcyclohexanone
- 2,3,5-Trimethylpyrazine
- 1-Tyrosine
- delta-Undercalactone
- gamma-Undecalactone
- Undecanal
- 2-Undecanone, 1
- 0-Undecenal
- Urea
- Valencene
- Valeraldehyde
- Valerian root extract, oil and powder
- Valeric ocid
- gamma-Valerolactone
- Valine
- Vanilla extract and oleoresin
- Vanillin
- Veratraldehyde
- Vetiver oil
- Vinegar
- Violet leaf absolute
- Walnut hull extract
- Water
- Wheat extract and flour
- Wild cherry bark extract
- Wine and wine sherry
- Xanthan gum
- 3,4-Xylenol
- Yeast

Chapter 4

Smoking's Immediate Effects On The Body

Many teenagers and adults think that there are no effects of smoking on their bodies until they reach middle age. Smoking-caused lung cancer, other cancers, heart disease, and stroke typically do not occur until years after a person's first cigarette. However, there are many serious harms from smoking that occur much sooner. In fact, smoking has numerous immediate health effects on the brain and on the respiratory, cardiovascular, gastrointestinal, immune, and metabolic systems. While these immediate effects do not all produce noticeable symptoms, most begin to damage the body with the first cigarette—sometimes irreversibly—and rapidly produce serious medical conditions and health consequences.

Rapid Addiction From Early Smoking

Many teenagers and younger children inaccurately believe that experimenting with smoking or even casual use will not lead to any serious dependency. In fact, the latest research shows that serious symptoms of addiction—such as having strong urges to smoke, feeling anxious or irritable, or having unsuccessfully tried to not smoke—can appear among youths within weeks or only days after occasional smoking first begins. The average smoker tries their first cigarette at age 12 and may be a regular smoker by age 14. Every day, more

About This Chapter: Text in this chapter is from "Smoking's Immediate Effects On The Body," reprinted with permission from the Campaign for Tobacco-Free Kids, © 2008. To view the complete document including references, visit www.tobaccofreekids.org.

than 3,500 kids try their first cigarette, and another 1,000 other kids under 18 years of age become new regular, daily smokers. Almost 90% of youths that smoke regularly report seriously strong cravings, and more than 70% of adolescent smokers have already tried and failed to quit smoking.

Immediate And Rapid Effects On The Brain

Part of the addictive power of nicotine comes from its direct effect on the brain. In addition to the well-understood chemical dependency, cigarette smokers also show evidence of a higher rate of behavioral problems and suffer the following immediate effects:

Increases Stress: Contrary to popular belief, smoking does not relieve stress. Studies have shown that on average, smokers have higher levels of stress than nonsmokers. The feelings of relaxation that smokers experience while they are smoking are actually a return to the normal unstressed state that nonsmokers experience all of the time.

Alters Brain Chemistry: When compared to nonsmokers, smokers brain cells, specifically brain cell receptors, have been shown to have fewer dopamine receptors. Brain cell receptors are molecules that sit on the outside of the cell interacting with the molecules that fit into the receptor, much like a lock and key.

Receptors (locks) are important because they guard and mediate the functions of the cell. For instance when the right molecule (key) comes along it unlocks the receptor, setting off a chain of events to perform a specific cell function. Specific receptors mediate different cell activities.

Smokers have fewer dopamine receptors, a specific cell receptor found in the brain that is believed to play a role in addiction. Dopamine is normally released naturally while engaging in certain behaviors like eating, drinking, and copulation. The release of dopamine is believed to give one a sense of reward. One of the leading hypothesis regarding the mechanism of addiction theorizes that nicotine exposure initially increases dopamine transmission, but subsequently decreases dopamine receptor function and number. The initial increase in dopamine activity from nicotine results initially in pleasant feelings for the smoker, but the subsequent decrease in dopamine leaves the smoker craving more cigarettes.

✤ It's A Fact!!

New animal studies have shown that brain chemistry and receptors may be altered early in the smoking process. Habitual smoking may continue to change brain chemistry, including decreasing dopamine receptors and thus yielding a more intense craving and risk of addiction. These brain chemistry changes may be permanent. In addition, because the role played by receptors in other cognitive functions, such as memory and intelligence, is unknown, how cigarette smoking affects other brain functions by altering brain chemistry is unknown.

Immediate And Rapid Effects On The Respiratory System

The respiratory system includes the passages from the nose and sinuses down into the smallest airways of the lungs. Because all of these spaces are in direct communication with one another, they can all be affected by tobacco smoke simultaneously.

Bronchospasm: This term refers to "airway irritability" or the abnormal tightening of the airways of the lungs. Bronchospasm makes airways smaller and leads to wheezing similar to that experienced by someone with asthma during an asthma attack. While smokers may not have asthma, they are susceptible to this type of reaction to tobacco smoke. An asthmatic who starts smoking can severely worsen his/her condition. Bronchospasm makes breathing more difficult, as the body tries to get more air into irritated lungs.

Increases Phlegm Production: The lungs produce mucus to trap chemical and toxic substances. Small "finger like" hairs, called cilia, coat the lung's airways and move rhythmically to clear this mucus from the lungs. Combined with coughing, this is usually an effective method of clearing the lungs of harmful substances. Tobacco smoke paralyzes these hairs, allowing mucus to collect in the lungs of the smoker. Cigarette smoke also promotes goblet cell growth resulting in an increase in mucus. More mucus is made with each breath of irritating tobacco and the smoker cannot easily clear the increased mucus.

Persistent Cough: Coughing is the body's natural response to clear irritants from the lungs. Without the help of cilia (above), a smoker is faced with the difficult task of clearing increased amounts of phlegm with cough alone. A persistent cough, while irritating, is the smoker's only defense against the harmful products of tobacco smoke.

Decreases Physical Performance: When the body is stressed or very active (for example, running, swimming, playing competitive sports), it requires that more oxygen be delivered to active muscles. The combination of bronchospasm and increased phlegm production result in airway obstruction and decreased lung function, leading to poor physical performance. In addition, smoking has been shown to stunt lung development in adolescent girls, limiting adult breathing capacity. Smoking not only limits one's current state of fitness, but can also restricts future physical potential.

☞ Remember!!

A smoker will likely have a persistent, annoying cough from the time they start smoking. A smoker who is not coughing is probably not doing an effective job of clearing his/her lungs of the harmful irritants found in tobacco smoke.

Immediate And Rapid Effects On The Cardiovascular System

The cardiovascular system includes the heart and all of the blood vessels that carry blood to and from the organs. Blood vessels include arteries, veins, and capillaries, which are all connected and work in unison with the lungs to deliver oxygen to the brain, heart, and other vital organs.

Adverse Lipid Profile: Lipids, a form of fat, are a source of energy for the body. Most people use this fat in its good form, called high-density lipoproteins, or HDLs. Some forms of fat, such as low-density lipoproteins (LDLs, triglycerides, and cholesterol) can be harmful to the body. These harmful forms have their greatest effects on blood vessels. If produced in excess or accumulated over time, they can stick to blood vessel walls and cause narrowing. Such narrowing can impair blood flow to the heart, brain and other organs, causing them to fail. Most bodies have a balance of good and bad fats. However, that is not the case for smokers. Nicotine increases the amount of bad fats (LDL, triglycerides, cholesterol) circulating in the blood vessels and decreases the amount of good fat (HDL) available. These silent effects begin immediately and greatly increase the risk for heart disease and stroke. In fact, smoking one-to-five cigarettes per day presents a significant risk for a heart attack.

Atherosclerosis: Atherosclerosis is a process in which fat and cholesterol form "plaques" and stick to the walls of an artery. These plaques reduce the blood's flow through the artery. While this process starts at a very young age (some children younger than one year of age already show some of the changes that lead to plaque formation) there are several factors that can accelerate atherosclerosis. Nicotine and other toxic substances from tobacco smoke are absorbed through the lungs into the blood stream and are circulated throughout the body. These substances damage the blood vessel walls, which allow plaques to form at a faster rate than they would in a nonsmoker. In this way, smoking increases the risk of heart disease by hastening atherosclerosis. In addition, a recent study in Japan showed a measurable decrease in the elasticity of the coronary arteries of nonsmokers after just 30 minutes of exposure to second-hand smoke.

Thrombosis: Thrombosis is a process that results in the formation of a clot inside a blood vessel. Normally, clots form inside blood vessels to stop bleeding, when vessels have been injured. However, components of tobacco smoke result in dangerously increased rates of clot formation. Smokers have elevated levels of thrombin, an enzyme that causes the blood to clot, after fasting, as well as a spike immediately after smoking. This process may result in blockage of blood vessels, stopping blood flow to vital organs. In addition, thrombosis especially occurs around sites of plaque formation (above).

Because of this abnormal tendency to clot, smokers with less severe heart disease, have more heart attacks than nonsmokers. In addition, sudden death is four times more likely to occur in young male cigarette smokers than in nonsmokers.

Constricts Blood Vessels: It has been shown that smoking, even light smoking, causes the body's blood vessels to constrict (vasoconstriction). Smoking does this by decreasing the nitric oxide (NO_2), which dilates blood vessels, and increasing the endothelin-1 (ET-1), which causes constriction of blood vessels. The net effect is constriction of blood vessels right after smoking and transient reduction in blood supply. Vasoconstriction may have immediate complications for certain persons, particularly individuals whose blood vessels are already narrowed by plaques (atherosclerosis), or partial blood clots, or individuals who are in a hypercoagulable state (have sickle cell disease). These individuals will be at increased risk of stroke or heart attack.

Increases Heart Rate: Heart rate is a measure of how fast your heart is pumping blood around your body. Young adult smokers have a resting heart rate of two to three beats per minute faster than the resting heart rate of young adult nonsmokers. Nicotine consumption increases a resting heart rate, as soon as 30 minutes after puffing; and the higher the nicotine consumption (through deep inhalation or increased number of cigarettes) the higher the heart rate. Smokers' hearts have to work harder than nonsmokers' hearts. A heart that is working harder is a heart that can tire-out faster and may result in an early heart attack or stroke.

Increases Blood Pressure: Blood pressure is a measure of tension upon the walls of arteries by blood. It is reported as a fraction, systolic over diastolic pressure. Systolic blood pressure is the highest arterial pressure reached during contraction of the heart. Diastolic blood pressure is the lowest pressure, found during the heart's relaxation phase. Nicotine consumption increases blood pressure. Older male smokers have been found to have higher systolic blood pressure than nonsmoking men do. Higher blood pressure requires that the heart pump harder in order to overcome the opposing pressure in the arteries. This increased work, much like that related to increased heart rate, can wear out a heart faster. The higher pressure can also cause organ damage where blood is filtered, such as in the kidneys.

Immediate And Rapid Effects On The Gastrointestinal System

The gastrointestinal system is responsible for digesting food, absorbing nutrients, and dispensing of waste products. It includes the mouth, esophagus, stomach, small and large intestines, and the anus. These continuous parts are all easily affected by tobacco smoke.

Gastroesophageal Reflux Disease: This disease includes symptoms of heartburn and acid regurgitation from the stomach. Normally the body prevents these occurrences by secreting a base to counteract digestive acids and by keeping the pathway between the esophagus (the tube between the mouth and stomach) and stomach tightly closed; except when the stomach is accepting food from above. The base smokers' bodies secrete is less neutralizing than nonsmokers and thus allows digestive acids a longer period of time to irritate the esophagus. Smokers also have an intermittent loosening of the muscle separating the esophagus and stomach, increasing the chance of stomach acid rising up to damage the esophagus. These immediate changes in base secretion and esophagus/stomach communication cause painful heartburn and result in an increased risk of long-term inflammation and dysfunction of the esophagus and stomach. Smoking also increases reflux of stomach contents into the esophagus and pharynx. Occurring regularly over time, this reflux may cause ulcerations of the lower esophagus, called Barrett's esophagus, to develop. Barrett's esophagus may develop into esophageal cancer, which has a poor prognosis in most patients.

Peptic Ulcer Disease: Peptic ulcers are self-digested holes extending into the muscular layers of the esophagus, stomach, and a portion of the small intestine. These ulcers form when excess acid is produced or when the protective inner layer of these structures is injured. Mucus is produced in the stomach to provide a protective barrier between stomach acid and cells of the stomach. Unlike in the lungs where mucus production is stimulated by cigarette smoke, mucous production in the stomach is inhibited. Peptic ulcers usually result from a failure of wound-healing due to outside factors, including tobacco smoke. Cigarette smoking increases acid exposure of the esophagus and stomach, while limiting neutralizing base production (above). Smoking also decreases blood flow to the inner layer of the esophagus, stomach and small intestine. In these ways, cigarette smoking immediately hinders gastrointestinal wound healing, which has been shown to result in peptic ulcer formation, when not treated. Peptic ulcers are terribly painful and treatment involves the long-term use of medications. Complications of peptic ulcers often require hospitalization and may be fatal secondary to excessive blood loss.

Periodontal Diseases: These occur when groups of bacteria are able to form colonies that cause infections and diseases of the mouth. Smoking quickly changes the blood supply, immune response, and healing mechanisms of the mouth, resulting in the rapid initiation and progression of infections. In this way, smoking makes the mouth more vulnerable to infections and allows the infections to become more severe. The bacterial plaques of smoking also cause gum inflammation and tooth decay. In addition, smoking increases tooth and bone loss and hastens deep gum pocket formation.

Halitosis: This is a fancy word for bad breath. Everybody knows that smoking makes individuals and everything around them smell bad. Bad breath, smelly hair and clothes, and yellow teeth are among the most immediate and unattractive effects of smoking.

Immediate And Rapid Effects On The Immune System

The immune system is the body's major defense against the outside world. It is a complicated system that involves several different types of cells that attack and destroy foreign substances. It begins in the parts of the body, which are in direct contact with the environment, such as the skin, ears, nose, mouth, stomach, and lungs. When these barriers become compromised, there are serious health consequences. Tobacco smoke weakens the immune system in a number of ways.

Otitis Media: This is inflammation of the middle ear. The middle ear is the space immediately behind the eardrum. It turns received vibrations into sound. The middle ear is very vulnerable to infection. Children exposed to environmental tobacco smoke (ETS) have more ear infections than those not exposed. Tobacco smoke disrupts the normal clearing mechanism of the ear canal, facilitating infectious organism entry into the body. The resulting middle ear infection can be very painful, as pressure and fluid build up in the ear. Continued exposure to tobacco smoke may result in persistent middle ear infections and eventually, hearing loss.

Sinusitis: Sinusitis is sinus inflammation. Sinuses are spaces in the skull that are in direct communication with the nose and mouth. They are important for warming and moisturizing inhaled air. The lining of the sinuses consists of the same finger-like hairs found in the lungs. These hairs clear mucus and foreign substances and are therefore critical in preventing mucus buildup and subsequent infection. Cigarette smoke slows or stops the movement of these hairs, resulting in inflammation and infection. Sinusitis can cause headaches, facial pain, tenderness, and swelling. It can also cause fever, cough, runny nose, sore throat, bad breath, and a decreased sense of smell.

☞ **Remember!!**

Sinusitis is more serious and requires a longer course of medical treatment than the common cold. Long-term smoke exposure can result in more frequent episodes and chronic cases of sinusitis, and the rate of sinusitis among smokers is high.

Rhinitis: This is an inflammation of the inner lining of the nasal passages and results in symptoms of sneezing, congestion, runny nose, and itchy eyes, ears, and nose. Similar to symptoms of the common cold, rhinitis may begin immediately in the regular smoker. Smoking causes rhinitis by damaging the same clearing mechanism involved in sinusitis (above). Rhinitis can cause sleep disturbances, activity limitations, irritability, moodiness, and decreased school performance. Smoking causes immediate and long-lasting rhinitis.

Pneumonia: Pneumonia is an inflammation of the lining of the lungs. This inflammation causes fluid to accumulate deep in the lung, making it an ideal region for bacterial growth. Pneumonia results in a persistent cough and difficulty breathing. A serious case of pneumonia often requires hospitalization. Smoking increases the body's susceptibility to the most common bacterial causes of pneumonia and is therefore a risk factor for pneumonia, regardless of age. Pneumonia, if left untreated, can lead to pus pocket formation, lung collapse, blood infection, and severe chest pain.

Immediate And Rapid Effects On The Metabolic System

Your metabolic system includes a complicated group of processes that break down foods and medicines into their components. Proteins, called enzymes, are responsible for this breakdown. The metabolic system involves many organs, especially those of the gastrointestinal tract.

Scurvy And Other Micronutrient Disorders: Micronutrients are dietary components necessary to maintain good health. These include vitamins, minerals, enzymes (above) and other elements that are critical to normal function. They must be consumed and absorbed in sufficient quantities to meet the body's needs. The daily requirement of these micronutrients changes naturally with age and can also be affected by environmental factors, including tobacco smoke. Smoking interferes with the absorption of a number of micronutrients, especially vitamins C, E, and folic acid that can result in deficiencies of these vitamins. A deficiency in Vitamin C can lead to scurvy which is a disease characterized by weakness, depression, inflamed gums, poor wound healing, and uncontrolled bleeding. Vitamin E deficiency may cause blood breakdown, eye disease, and irreversible nerve problems of the hands, feet, and spinal cord. Folic acid deficiency may result in long-lasting anemia, diarrhea, and tongue swelling.

Oxidative Damage: Oxidants are active particles that are byproducts of normal chemical processes that are constantly underway inside the body. Their formation is called oxidation. These particles are usually found and destroyed by antioxidants, including vitamins A, C, and E. The balance of oxidation and anti-oxidation is critical to health. When oxidation overwhelms anti-oxidation, harmful consequences occur. Oxidants directly damage cells and change genetic material, likely contributing to the development of cancer, heart disease, and cataracts. Oxidants also speed up blood vessel damage due to atherosclerosis (above), which is a known risk factor for heart disease. Because smoking increases the number of circulating oxidants, it also increases the consumption of existing antioxidants. This increase in antioxidant consumption reduces the levels of antioxidants such as alpha-tocopherol, the active form of vitamin E. Smoking immediately causes oxidant stress in blood while the antioxidant potential is reduced because of this stress. This dangerous imbalance cannot be neutralized and results in immediate cell, gene, and blood vessel damage. In addition, a National Cancer Institute study found that beta-carotene supplements, which contain precursors of vitamin A, modestly increase the incidence of lung cancer and overall mortality in cigarette smokers.

Immediate And Rapid Effects On Drug Interactions

Drug breakdown, or metabolism, is important to drug effectiveness and safety. Medicines are naturally broken down into their components by enzymes. Factors that effect drug metabolism effect drug function. Factors that speed up drug metabolism decrease drug exposure time and reduce the circulating concentrations of the drug, which compromises the effectiveness of the prescription. Conversely, factors that slow down drug metabolism increase the circulating time and concentration of the drug, allowing the drug to be present at harmful levels.

Tobacco smoke interferes with many medications by both of these mechanisms. For example, the components of tobacco smoke hasten the breakdown of some blood-thinners, antidepressants, and anti-seizure medications; and tobacco smoke also decreases the effectiveness of certain sedatives, painkillers, heart, ulcer, and asthma medicines.

Especially Vulnerable Populations

Asthmatics: Mainstream or environmental tobacco smoke (ETS) exacerbates asthma symptoms in known asthmatics. In addition, some studies have shown a link between ETS in childhood and a higher prevalence of asthma in adulthood.

Infants and Children: Infants and children exposed to environmental tobacco smoke (ETS) are at increased risk for death and disease. Mothers who smoke during pregnancy are known to have low birth-weight babies. In breastfeeding women who smoke, there is a decrease in maternal milk production and less weight gain in the exposed infant. In addition, infants whose mothers smoke have an increased risk of sudden infant death syndrome (SIDS), and their overall perinatal mortality rate is 25–56% higher than those infants of mothers who choose not to smoke. Children exposed to ETS are at increased risk of many infections, most commonly middle ear and respiratory infections, and thus require more doctor visits and hospital stays.

Sickle Cell Patients: Patients with sickle cell anemia who smoke are known to have increased incidence of acute chest syndrome. Acute chest syndrome is a condition that presents with severe chest pain and is a life-threatening emergency.

☞ Remember!!

While some of these effects are wholly or partially reversible upon quitting smoking, research has shown that many are not. Quitting smoking provides enormous health benefits, but some smoking-caused damage simply cannot be reversed. Moreover, many of the effects outlined here can cause considerable harm to kids and others soon after they begin smoking and well before they become long-term smokers.

Chapter 5

The Process Of Nicotine Addiction

Tobacco use is an addiction. Nicotine is a drug. It can affect people in many different ways. It can be hard to quit for several reasons.

Any addiction has three major areas of dependence:

- Physical, also known as chemical

- Emotional, also called psychological

- Social or behavioral, also known as habit

Physical Or Chemical Dependence

- When you use tobacco, nicotine travels to your brain and attaches to nicotine receptors. The nicotine receptors cause certain chemical reactions in your brain leaving you with a sense of pleasure and relaxation.

- Your body creates more nicotine receptors as you become more physically dependent to nicotine. This is called up regulation.

- When you try to quit smoking or using smokeless tobacco, your brain continues to crave the nicotine. This can make it harder to quit.

About This Chapter: Text in this chapter is from "The Process of Nicotine Addiction," © 2009 Health System Nursing, The Ohio State University Medical Center. All rights reserved. Reprinted with permission. For additional information, visit http://medicalcenter .osu.edu/patientcare/patient_education.

✤ It's A Fact!!
How does tobacco affect the brain?

Cigarettes and other forms of tobacco—including cigars, pipe tobacco, snuff, and chewing tobacco—contain the addictive drug nicotine. Nicotine is readily absorbed into the bloodstream when a tobacco product is chewed, inhaled, or smoked. A typical smoker will take ten puffs on a cigarette over a period of five minutes that the cigarette is lit. Thus, a person who smokes about one and a half packs (30 cigarettes) daily gets 300 "hits" of nicotine each day.

Upon entering the bloodstream, nicotine immediately stimulates the adrenal glands to release the hormone epinephrine (adrenaline). Epinephrine stimulates the central nervous system and increases blood pressure, respiration, and heart rate. Glucose is released into the blood while nicotine suppresses insulin output from the pancreas, which means that smokers have chronically elevated blood sugar levels.

Like cocaine, heroin, and marijuana, nicotine increases levels of the neurotransmitter dopamine, which affects the brain pathways that control reward and pleasure. For many tobacco users, long-term brain changes induced by continued nicotine exposure result in addiction—a condition of compulsive drug seeking and use, even in the face of negative consequences. Studies suggest that additional compounds in tobacco smoke, such as acetaldehyde, may enhance nicotine's effects on the brain. A number of studies indicate that adolescents are especially vulnerable to these effects and may be more likely than adults to develop an addiction to tobacco.

When an addicted user tries to quit, he or she experiences withdrawal symptoms including powerful cravings for tobacco, irritability, difficulty paying attention, sleep disturbances, and increased appetite. Treatments can help smokers manage these symptoms and improve the likelihood of successfully quitting.

Source: Excerpted from "NIDA InfoFacts: Cigarettes and Other Tobacco Products," National Institute on Drug Abuse, June 2009.

- Your body may go through withdrawal until the number of nicotine receptors returns to the amount there were before you started to use tobacco. Withdrawal often lasts seven to 30 days.

- Signs of withdrawal may include:

  - Depressed mood;

  - Problems sleeping;

  - Being irritable, frustrated or angry;

  - Feeling anxious or nervous;

  - Problems concentrating;

  - Being restless;

  - Slowed heart beat;

  - Increased appetite or weight gain.

- Other facts about nicotine in your body:

  - Most smokers inhale one to two milligrams of nicotine from each cigarette. That means the brain of a pack a day smoker gets 200 hits on nicotine each day.

  - Tobacco smoke contains more than 50 known cancer causing agents, although nicotine is not thought to cause cancer.

  - Nicotine goes into your lungs and is picked up by the oxygen rich blood there. It is then carried to all parts of your brain and body as your heart pumps.

  - Nicotine in cigarette smoke reaches the brain in 10 seconds.

  - Nicotine causes a release of dopamine in your brain's reward center. Some behaviors around tobacco use may also have this effect.

Emotional Or Psychological Dependence

Many times, using tobacco becomes a way to deal with certain situations and emotions like stress, anger, sadness, or loneliness. Since nicotine produces feelings of pleasure, many people use tobacco to cope during tough times.

Tobacco is always there for you. When you quit tobacco, it may feel like you are losing your best friend. Developing new coping skills is an important part of the quitting process.

♣ It's A Fact!!
Genes And Addiction

Most of the 44.5 million American adults who smoke cigarettes would prefer not to. Why do so many would-be quitters fail, even with the help of stop-smoking interventions like nicotine replacement? Why, for that matter, do people become addicted to smoking in the first place? The answers lie partly in our genes.

Researchers at the National Institute on Drug Abuse (NIDA) in collaboration with Perlegen Sciences, Inc., a private company, recently completed a search of the entire human genome for differences between individuals who are nicotine-dependent and those who smoked but never became dependent. Their target: single nucleotide polymorphisms (SNPs), locations on the genome where individuals differ by just one chemical unit in the makeup of their DNA. From 2.2 million known SNPs, researchers have identified roughly 40 to 80 that are highly correlated with nicotine addiction.

Once researchers link an SNP statistically to drug abuse, the question becomes: Does the gene do anything that might explain why people with one of its forms are more vulnerable to drugs than people with another? Some of the genes researchers have implicated in addiction affect the dopamine reward circuit. Others involve neurotransmitter systems and neural pathways not previously known to figure in smoking's effects. Researchers will use techniques such as brain imaging to correlate genetic differences with differences in brain structure or function and psychological tests to match them to behavior. Findings from the genome exploration may ultimately yield novel, more effective interventions.

Genetic variations can only partly explain why people become addicted to nicotine: A person's genetic makeup, experiences, and surroundings all combine to determine whether he or she will smoke and, if so, how difficult quitting will be.

Source: Excerpted from "Genes and Smoking," by Nora D. Volkow, MD, National Institute on Drug Abuse, April 2007.

Social Or Behavioral Dependence Or Habit

A habit is a pattern of learned behavior that develops after many repetitions. A habit can become deeply rooted in as little as three weeks.

Most tobacco users develop a habit of using around certain times or activities, such as after meals or around other users.

Smoking is a learned behavior. You need to unlearn the behavior in order to quit. One way to break the habit can be to track your tobacco use to see what activities or times of day you are most likely to use tobacco. These are called your triggers. This can help you create your own quit plan.

If you have questions about quitting tobacco use, call the Ohio State University Medical Center (OSUMC) Tobacco Treatment Center toll free at 866-504-0561.

Talk to your doctor or others on your health care team if you have questions. You may request more written information from the Library for Health Information at 614-293-3707 or e-mail: health-info@osu.edu.

Chapter 6

Young People And Tobacco: A Statistical Review

Tobacco Use And The Health Of Young People

Tobacco Use By Young People

- Each day in the United States, approximately 4,000 adolescents aged 12–17 try their first cigarette.

- Each year cigarette smoking accounts for approximately one of every five deaths, or about 438,000 people. Cigarette smoking results in 5.5 million years of potential life lost in the United States annually.

- Although the percentage of high school students who smoke has declined in recent years, rates remain high: 20% of high school students report current cigarette use (smoked cigarettes on at least one day during the 30 days before the survey).

- Fifty percent of high school students have ever tried cigarette smoking, even one or two puffs.

About This Chapter: Text in this chapter begins with "Tobacco Use: Tobacco Use and the Health of Young People," National Center for Chronic Disease Prevention and Health Promotion, Centers for Disease Control and Prevention (CDC), July 11, 2008. It continues with "Youth and Tobacco Use: Current Estimates," CDC, May 29, 2009.

- Fourteen percent of high school students have smoked a whole cigarette before age 13.

- Nearly 8% of high school students (13% of male and 2% of female students) used smokeless tobacco (for example, chewing tobacco, snuff, or dip), on at least one day during the 30 days before the survey. Adolescents who use smokeless tobacco are more likely than nonusers to become cigarette smokers.

- Fourteen percent of high school students smoked cigars, cigarillos, or little cigars on at least one day during the 30 days before the survey.

Table 6.1. Prevalence of Current Cigarette Use Among High School Students, 2007

Racial/Ethnic Group	Male	Female	Overall
Black (Non-Hispanic)	14.9 %	8.4 %	11.6 %
Hispanic	18.7 %	14.6 %	16.7 %
White (Non-Hispanic)	23.8 %	22.5 %	23.2 %

Health Effects Of Tobacco Use By Young People

- Cigarette smoking by young people leads to immediate and serious health problems including respiratory and nonrespiratory effects, addiction to nicotine, and the associated risk of other drug use.

- Smoking at an early age increases the risk of lung cancer. For most smoking-related cancers, the risk rises as the individual continues to smoke.

- Cigarette smoking causes heart disease, stroke, chronic lung disease, and cancers of the lung, mouth, pharynx, esophagus, and bladder.

- Use of smokeless tobacco causes cancers of the mouth, pharynx and esophagus; gum recession; and an increased risk for heart disease and stroke.

- Smoking cigars increases the risk of oral, laryngeal, esophageal, and lung cancers.

✤ It's A Fact!!
Are there gender differences in tobacco smoking?

Several avenues of research now indicate that men and women differ in their smoking behaviors. For instance, women smoke fewer cigarettes per day, tend to use cigarettes with lower nicotine content, and do not inhale as deeply as men. However, it is unclear whether this is due to differences in sensitivity to nicotine or other factors that affect women differently, such as social factors or the sensory aspects of smoking.

The number of smokers in the United States declined in the 1970s and 1980s, remained relatively stable throughout the 1990s, and declined further through the early 2000s. Because this decline in smoking was greater among men than women, the prevalence of smoking is only slightly higher for men today than it is for women.

Several factors appear to be contributing to this narrowing gender gap, including women being less likely than men to quit. Large-scale smoking cessation trials show that women are less likely to initiate quitting and may be more likely to relapse if they do quit. In cessation programs using nicotine replacement methods, such as the patch or gum, the nicotine does not seem to reduce craving as effectively for women as for men. Other factors that may contribute to women's difficulty with quitting are that withdrawal may be more intense for women or that women are more concerned about weight gain.

Although postcessation weight gain is typically modest (about 5–10 pounds), concerns about this may be an obstacle to treatment success. In fact, research conducted by the National Institute on Drug Abuse (NIDA) has found that when women's weight concerns were addressed during cognitive-behavioral therapy, they were more successful at quitting than women who were in a program designed only to attenuate postcessation weight gain. Other NIDA researchers have found that medications used for smoking cessation, such as bupropion and naltrexone, can also attenuate postcessation weight gain and could become an additional strategy for enhancing treatment success. It is important for treatment professionals to be aware that standard regimens may have to be adjusted to compensate for gender differences in nicotine sensitivity and in other related factors that contribute to continued smoking.

Source: Excerpted from "Research Report Series: Tobacco Addiction," National Institute on Drug Abuse, June 2009.

Nicotine Addiction Among Young People

- The younger people begin smoking cigarettes, the more likely they are to become strongly addicted to nicotine. Young people who try to quit suffer the same nicotine withdrawal symptoms as adults who try to quit.

- Several studies have found nicotine to be addictive in ways similar to heroin, cocaine, and alcohol. Of all addictive behaviors, cigarette smoking is the one most likely to become established during adolescence.

- Among high school students who are current smokers, 50% have tried to quit smoking cigarettes during the 12 months before the survey.

Tobacco Sales And Promoting To Youth

- All states have laws making it illegal to sell cigarettes to anyone under the age of 18, yet 16% of students under the age of 18 who currently smoke cigarettes reported they usually obtained their own cigarettes by buying them in a store or gas station during the 30 days before the survey.

- Cigarette companies spent more than $15.2 billion in 2003 to promote their products. Children and teenagers constitute the majority of all new smokers, and the industry's advertising and promotion campaigns often have special appeal to these young people.

- Eighty-three percent of young smokers (aged 12–17) choose the three most heavily advertised brands.

Health Effects Of Secondhand Smoke In Youth

- An estimated 10–11 million youth aged 12–18 live in a household with at least one smoker, and over six million are exposed to secondhand smoke daily.

- Those most affected by secondhand smoke are children. Because their bodies are still developing, exposure to the poisons in secondhand smoke puts children in danger of severe respiratory diseases and may hinder the growth of their lungs.

- Secondhand smoke exposure during childhood and adolescence may contribute to new cases of asthma or worsen existing asthma.

There is no risk-free level of secondhand smoke exposure. Even brief exposure can be dangerous.

Youth And Tobacco Use: Current Estimates

Cigarette Smoking

- In 2007, 20% of high school students in the United States were current cigarette smokers—approximately 19% of females and 21% of males.

- Among racial and ethnic subgroups, approximately 23% of white, 17% of Hispanic, and 12% of African American high school students were current cigarette smokers in 2007.

- In 2006, approximately 6% of middle school students in this country were current cigarette smokers, with estimates of 6% for females and 6% for males.

- Among racial and ethnic subgroups, approximately 7% of white, 7% of Hispanic, 6% of African American, and 3% of Asian American middle school students were current cigarette smokers in 2006.

- Each day in the United States, approximately 3,600 young people between the ages of 12 and 17 years initiate cigarette smoking, and an estimated 1,100 young people become daily cigarette smokers.

- More than 13% of high school students were current cigar smokers in 2007, with estimates higher for males (19%) than for females (8%).

- Nationally, an estimated 4% of all middle school students were current smokeless tobacco users in 2006, with estimates slightly higher for males (5%) than for females (3%).

- An estimated 13% of males in high school were current smokeless tobacco users in 2007.

- An estimated 4% of males in middle school were current smokeless tobacco users in 2006.

- In 2006, approximately 3% of high school students were current users of bidis; bidi use among males was (3%) and (2%) for females. Among middle school students, approximately 2% were bidi users, with estimates of 2% for males and 2% for females.

✤ It's A Fact!!
Tobacco Facts

Tobacco is one of the strongest cancer-causing agents. Tobacco use is associated with a number of different cancers, including lung cancer, as well as with chronic lung diseases and cardiovascular diseases.

Cigarette smoking remains the leading preventable cause of death in the United States, causing an estimated 438,000 deaths—or about one out of every five—each year.

In the United States, approximately 38,000 deaths each year are caused by exposure to secondhand smoke.

Lung cancer is the leading cause of cancer death among both men and women in the United States, with 90% of lung cancer deaths among men and approximately 80% of lung cancer deaths among women attributed to smoking.

Smoking also increases the risk of many other types of cancer, including cancers of the throat, mouth, pancreas, kidney, bladder, and cervix.

People who smoke are up to six times more likely to suffer a heart attack than nonsmokers, and the risk increases with the number of cigarettes smoked. Smoking also causes most cases of chronic obstructive lung disease, which includes bronchitis and emphysema.

In 2007, approximately 19.8% of U.S. adults were cigarette smokers.

Twenty-three percent of high school students and 8% of middle school students in this country are current cigarette smokers.

In the United States, an estimated 8% of high school students are current smokeless tobacco users. An estimated 3% of middle school students in this country are current smokeless tobacco users.

Source: From "Tobacco Facts," National Cancer Institute, November 24, 2008. The complete text of this document, including references, can be found online at www.cancer.gov/cancertopics/tobacco/statisticssnapshot.

Factors Associated With Tobacco Use Among Youth

- Some factors associated with youth tobacco use include low socio-economic status, use and approval of tobacco use by peers or siblings, smoking by parents or guardians, accessibility, availability and price of tobacco products, a perception that tobacco use is normative, lack of parental support or involvement, low levels of academic achievement, lack of skills to resist influences to tobacco use, lower self-image or self-esteem, belief in functional benefits of tobacco use, and lack of self-efficacy to refuse offers of tobacco.

- Tobacco use in adolescence is associated with many other health risk behaviors, including high-risk sexual behavior and use of alcohol or other drugs.

Chapter 7

Global Trends In Tobacco Use

Although people have used tobacco for centuries, cigarettes did not appear in mass-manufactured form until the 19th century. Since then, the practice of cigarette smoking has spread worldwide on a massive scale. Today, about one in three adults, or 1.1 billion people, smoke. Of these, about 80% live in low- and middle-income countries. Partly because of growth in the adult population, and partly because of increased consumption, the total number of smokers is expected to reach about 1.6 billion by 2025.

In the past, tobacco was often chewed, or smoked in various kinds of pipes. While these practices persist, they are declining. Manufactured cigarettes and various types of hand-rolled cigarette such as bidis—common in Southeast Asia and India—now account for up to 85% of all tobacco consumed worldwide. Cigarette smoking appears to pose much greater dangers to health than earlier forms of tobacco use. This report therefore focuses on manufactured cigarettes and bidis.

About This Chapter: Text in this chapter is excerpted from *Curbing the Epidemic: Governments and the Economics of Tobacco Control*, ©1999 The World Bank (www.worldbank.org). Reprinted with permission of The World Bank via Copyright Clearance Center. Despite the older date of this document, the information is still useful for readers interested in information about the worldwide spread of tobacco use.

Rising Consumption In Low-Income And Middle-Income Countries

The populations of the low- and middle-income countries have been increasing their cigarette consumption since about 1970 (see Figure 7.1). The per capita consumption in these countries climbed steadily between 1970 and 1990, although the upward trend may have slowed a little since the early 1990s.

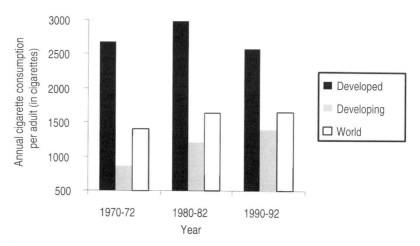

Source: World Health Organization. 1997. *Tobacco or Health: a Global Status Report.* Geneva, Switzerland.

Figure 7.1. *Smoking is increasing in the developing world, trends in per capita adult cigarette consumption.*

While the practice of smoking has become more prevalent among men in low- and middle-income countries, it has been in overall decline among men in the high-income countries during the same period. For example, more than 55% of men in the United States smoked at the peak of consumption in the mid-20th century, but the proportion had fallen to 28% by the mid-1990s. Per capita consumption for the populations of the high-income countries as a whole also has dropped. However, among certain groups in these countries, such as teenagers and young women, the proportion who smoke has grown in the 1990s. Overall, then, the smoking epidemic is spreading from its original focus, among men in high-income countries, to women in high-in-come countries and men in low-income regions.

In recent years, international trade agreements have liberalized global trade in many goods and services. Cigarettes are no exception. The removal of trade barriers tends to introduce greater competition that results in lower prices, greater advertising and promotion, and other activities that stimulate demand. One study concluded that, in four Asian economies that opened their markets in response to U.S. trade pressure during the 1980s (Japan, South Korea, Taiwan, and Thailand) consumption of cigarettes per person was almost 10% higher in 1991 than it would have been if these markets had remained closed. An econometric model developed for this report concludes that increased trade liberalization contributed significantly to increases in cigarette consumption, particularly in the low and middle-income countries.

Regional Patterns In Smoking

Data on the number of smokers in each region have been compiled by the World Health Organization using more than 80 separate studies. For the purpose of this report, these data have been used to estimate the prevalence of smoking in each of the seven World Bank country groupings. As Table 7.1 shows, there are wide variations between regions and, in particular, in the prevalence of smoking among women in different regions. For example, in Eastern Europe and Central Asia (mainly the former socialist economies), 59% of men and 26% of women smoked in 1995, more than in any other region. Yet in East Asia and the Pacific, where the prevalence of male smoking is equally high, at 59%, just 4% of women were smokers.

Smoking And Socioeconomic Status

Historically, as incomes rose within populations, the number of people who smoked rose too. In the earlier decades of the smoking epidemic in high-income countries, smokers were more likely to be affluent than poor. But in the past three to four decades, this pattern appears to have been reversed, at least among men, for whom data are widely available.

✤ It's A Fact!!
Research into women's smoking patterns is much more limited. Where women have been smoking for decades, the relationship between socioeconomic status and smoking is similar to that seen in men, Elsewhere, more reliable information is needed before conclusions can be drawn.

Table 7.1. Regional Patterns of Smoking. Estimated smoking prevalence by gender and number of smokers in population aged 15 or more, by World Bank region, 1995

World Bank Region	Smoking prevalence (%)			Total smokers	
					(% of all
	Males	Females	Overall	(millions)	smokers)
East Asia and Pacific	59	4	32	401	35
Eastern Europe and Central Asia	59	26	41	148	13
Latin America and Caribbean	40	21	30	95	8
Middle East and North Africa	44	5	25	40	3
South Asia (cigarettes)	20	1	11	86	8
South Asia (bidis)	20	3	12	96	8
Sub-Saharan Africa	33	10	21	67	6
Low/Middle Income	49	9	29	933	82
High Income	39	22	30	209	18
World	47	12	29	1,142	100

Note: Numbers have been rounded.

Source: Author's calculations based on World Health Organization. 1997. *Tobacco or Health: A Global Status Report.* Geneva, Switzerland

Affluent men in the high-income countries have increasingly abandoned tobacco, whereas poorer men have not done so. For example, in Norway, the percentage of men with high incomes who smoked fell from 75% in 1955 to 28% in 1990. Over the same period, the proportion of men on low incomes who smoked declined much less steeply, from 60% in 1955 to 48% in 1990. Today, in most high-income countries, there are significant differences in the prevalence of smoking between different socioeconomic groups. In the United Kingdom, for instance, only 10% of women and 12% of men in the highest socioeconomic group are smokers; in the lowest socioeconomic groups the corresponding figures are threefold greater: 35% and 40%. The same inverse relationship is found between education levels—a marker for socioeconomic status—and smoking. In general, individuals who have received little or no education are more likely to smoke than those who are more educated.

Until recently, it was thought that the situation in low- and middle-income countries was different. However, the most recent research concludes that here too, men of low socioeconomic status are more likely to smoke than those of high socioeconomic status. Educational level is a clear determinant of smoking in Chennai, India (Figure 7.2). Studies in Brazil, China, South Africa, Vietnam, and several Central American nations confirm this pattern.

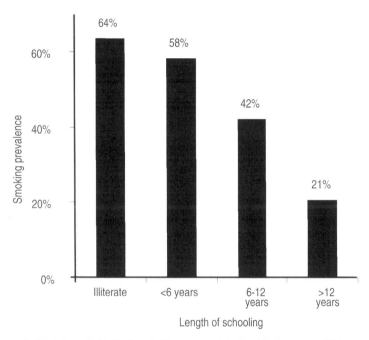

Source: Gajalakshmi, C. K., P. Jha, S. Nguyen, and A. Yurekli. *Patterns of Tobacco Use, and Health Consequences.* Background paper.

Figure 7.2. *Smoking is more common among the less educated: Smoking prevalence among men in Chennai (India), by education levels.*

While it is thus clear that the prevalence of smoking is higher among the poor and less educated worldwide, there are fewer data on the number of cigarettes smoked daily by different socioeconomic groups. In high-income countries, with some exceptions, poor and less educated men smoke more cigarettes per day than richer, more educated men. While it might have been expected that poor men in low- and middle-income countries would smoke fewer cigarettes than affluent men, the available data indicate that, in general, smokers with low levels of education consume equal or slightly larger numbers of cigarettes than those with high levels of education. An important exception is India, where, not surprisingly, smokers with college-level education status tend to consume more cigarettes, which are relatively more expensive, while smokers with low levels of education status consume larger numbers of the inexpensive bidis.

Age And The Uptake Of Smoking

It is unlikely that individuals who avoid starting to smoke in adolescence or young adulthood will ever become smokers. Nowadays, the overwhelming majority of smokers start before age 25, often in childhood or adolescence; in the high-income countries, eight out of 10 begin in their teens. In middle-income and low-income countries for which data are available, it appears that most smokers

---

✤ It's A Fact!!
How many young people take up smoking each day?

Individuals who start to smoke at a young age are likely to become heavy smokers, and are also at increased risk of dying from smoking-related diseases in later life. It is therefore important to know how many children and young people take up smoking daily. We attempt here to answer this question.

We used (1) World Bank data on the number of children and adolescents, male and female, who reached age 20 in 1995, for each World Bank region, and (2) data from the World Health Organization on the prevalence of smokers in all age groups up to the age of 30 in each of these regions. For an upper estimate, we assumed that the number of young people who take up smoking every day is a product of (1) times (2) per region, for each gender. For a lower estimate, we reduced this by region-specific estimates for the number of smokers who start after the age of 30.

start by the early twenties, but the trend is toward younger ages. For example, in China between 1984 and 1996, there was a significant increase in the number of young men aged between 15 and 19 years who took up smoking. A similar decline in the age of starting has been observed in the high-income countries.

Global Patterns Of Quitting

While there is evidence that smoking begins in youth worldwide, the proportion of smokers who quit appears to vary sharply between high-income countries and the rest of the world, at least to date. In environments of steadily increased knowledge about the health effects of tobacco, the prevalence of smoking has gradually fallen, and a significant number of former smokers have accumulated over the decades. In most high-income countries, about 30% of the male population are former smokers. In contrast, only 2% of Chinese men had quit in 1993, only 5% of Indian males at around the same period, and only 10% of Vietnamese males had quit in 1997.

We made three conservative assumptions: first, that there have been minimal changes over time in the average age of uptake. There have been recent downward trends in the age of uptake in young Chinese men, but assuming little change means that, if anything, our figures are underestimates. Second, we focused on regular smokers, excluding the much larger number of children who would try smoking but not become regular smokers. Third, we assumed that, for those young people who become regular smokers, quitting before adulthood is rare. While the number of adolescent regular smokers who quit is substantial in high-income countries, in low- and middle-income countries it is currently very low.

With these assumptions, we calculated that the number of children and young people taking up smoking ranges from 14,000 to 15,000 per day in the high-income countries as a whole. For middle- and low-income countries, the estimated numbers range from 68,000 to 84,000. This means that every day, worldwide, there are between 82,000 and 99,000 young people starting to smoke and risking rapid addiction to nicotine. These figures are consistent with existing estimates for individual high-income countries.

Chapter 8

Facts About Tobacco Advertising

Advertising Affects Tobacco Use

The tobacco industry spends billions of dollars each year to market its products. The industry uses a mix of advertising, promotion and sponsorship tactics to directly affect tobacco use and attitudes related to tobacco. Tobacco advertising, promotion and sponsorship:

- Promote tobacco use as customary and glamorous;

- Are deceptive and misleading;

- Weaken public health campaigns;

- Target specific populations such as women, youth, and minority groups.

Increase tobacco consumption by:

- Attracting new tobacco users;

- Increasing the amount of consumption among current smokers;

- Reducing a smoker's willingness to quit;

- Encouraging former smokers to start smoking again.

About This Chapter: Text in this chapter is excerpted from "Tobacco Advertising, Promotion and Sponsorship," reprinted with permission from the Campaign for Tobacco-Free Kids, © 2008. To view the complete document including references, visit www.tobacco freekids.org.

☞ Remember!!

Through advertising of its products, the tobacco industry tries to create an environment in which tobacco use is familiar and socially acceptable, and the warnings about its health consequences are undermined.

Comprehensive Bans Reduce Tobacco Use

Comprehensive bans, which prohibit the use of all marketing strategies by the tobacco industry, reduce tobacco use among people of all income and educational levels. Partial advertising bans are less effective, in part, because the tobacco industry switches its marketing efforts to unrestricted outlets when bans are not comprehensive.

- A study of 22 developed countries found that comprehensive bans reduced tobacco consumption by 6.3%.

- A study of 102 countries showed that in countries with partial bans consumption only decreased by 1% compared with almost 9% in countries with comprehensive bans.

- A study of 30 developing countries found partial bans were associated with a 13.6% reduction in per capita consumption, compared to 23.5% in countries with comprehensive bans.

The World Health Organization Framework Convention On Tobacco Control Requires Comprehensive Bans

The Framework Convention on Tobacco Control (FCTC), the world's first global public health treaty, establishes a policy framework aimed to reduce the devastating health, economic, and social impacts of tobacco. Article 13 of the FCTC requires parties to implement and enforce a comprehensive ban on tobacco advertising, promotion and sponsorship within five years of ratifying the FCTC.

Tobacco advertising and promotion is defined in the FCTC as "any form of commercial communication, recommendation or action with the aim, effect or likely effect of promoting a tobacco product either directly or indirectly."

Examples include:

- Broadcast, print and outdoor advertising;
- Point of sale advertising;
- Various sales and /or distribution arrangements with retailers for product placement, sales promotions and discounts;
- Product packaging;
- Advertising on the internet;
- Use of tobacco brand names, logos, or visual brand identities on non-tobacco products, activities, or events;
- Placement of tobacco products or tobacco use in the entertainment media.

Sponsorship is defined in the FCTC, as "any form of contribution to any event, activity or individual with aim, effect or likely effect of promoting a tobacco product or tobacco use either directly or indirectly."

Examples include:

- Sports;
- Cultural events;
- Concerts;
- School programs;
- Corporate social responsibility activities such as youth prevention initiatives and charitable contributions to public and private organizations.

Components Of A Comprehensive Ban

Legislation for a comprehensive ban on tobacco advertising, promotion and sponsorship must:

- Be complete and apply to all direct and indirect marketing and promotional strategies. In countries with constitutional limits that prevent the adoption of comprehensive bans, policies, at a minimum, should require health warnings on all forms of advertising, promotion and sponsorships, and ban all forms of false, misleading or deceptive advertising.

- Be broadly written to cover all forms of advertising, promotion and sponsorship. If examples are included in the legislation, it should be clear that they are provided for illustrative purposes only and are not meant to limit the comprehensive ban in any way.

- Undergo periodic review and amendment to address new marketing tactics developed by the industry.

- Cover all entities that engage or participate in tobacco advertising, promotion and sponsorship activities, such as media outlets and advertising firms.

- Cover cross-border advertising, promotion and sponsorship originating within a nation's territory.

- Include clear enforcement mechanisms to ensure the laws are effectively implemented.

Key Messages

- Tobacco advertising, promotion and sponsorship encourage people, especially youth, to use tobacco, encourage tobacco users to use more, decrease users' motivation to quit, and encourage quitters to relapse.

- A comprehensive ban on advertising, promotion and sponsorship reduces tobacco use; partial bans have limited or no effect on tobacco consumption.

> ✤ **It's A Fact!!**
> **Global Progress On Comprehensive Bans**
>
> Countries have the right to restrict the marketing of harmful products to protect the public's health. Countries which ban or restrict tobacco advertising, promotion and sponsorship, include: all European Union countries; Australia; New Zealand; South Africa; and Thailand.

- Parties to the FCTC are required to implement comprehensive bans on tobacco advertising, promotion and sponsorships within five years of ratifying the FCTC as a part of an effective set of tobacco control policies.

Chapter 9

Tobacco Company Marketing To Kids

From the 1950s to the present, different defendants, at different times and using different methods, have intentionally marketed to young people under the age of twenty-one in order to recruit "replacement smokers" to ensure the economic future of the tobacco industry. (U.S. District Court Judge Gladys Kessler Final Opinion, United States v. Philip Morris)

The major cigarette companies, alone, now spend about $13.1 billion per year (or more than $35.9 million every day) to promote their products; and many of their marketing efforts directly reach kids. In fact, cigarette company spending to market their deadly products increased by more than 95% from1998 to 2005 (the most recent year for which complete data is available). Moreover, tobacco industry documents, research on the effect of the cigarette companies' marketing efforts on kids, and the opinions of advertising experts combine to reveal the intent and the success of the industry's efforts to attract new smokers from the ranks of children.

Tobacco Industry Statements And Actions

Numerous internal tobacco industry documents, revealed in the various tobacco lawsuits, show that the tobacco companies have perceived kids as young as 13 years of age as a key market, studied the smoking habits of kids,

About This Chapter: The text in this chapter is excerpted from "Tobacco Company Marketing To Kids," reprinted with permission from the Campaign for Tobacco-Free Kids, 2008. To view the complete document including references, visit www.tobaccofreekids.org.

and developed products and marketing campaigns aimed at them. As an RJR Tobacco document put it, "Many manufacturers have 'studied' the 14–20 market in hopes of uncovering the 'secret' of the instant popularity some brands enjoy to the almost exclusion of others… Creating a 'fad' in this market can be a great bonanza." The following are just a few of the many more internal company quotes about marketing to kids:

Philip Morris: "Today's teenager is tomorrow's potential regular customer, and the overwhelming majority of smokers first begin to smoke while still in their teens…The smoking patterns of teenagers are particularly important to Philip Morris."

RJ Reynolds: "Evidence is now available to indicate that the 14–18 year old group is an increasing segment of the smoking population. RJR-T must soon establish a successful new brand in this market if our position in the industry is to be maintained in the long term."

Brown & Williamson: "Kool's stake in the 16- to 25-year-old population segment is such that the value of this audience should be accurately weighted and reflected in current media programs… all magazines will be reviewed to see how efficiently they reach this group."

Lorillard Tobacco: "[T]he base of our business is the high school student."

U.S. Tobacco: "Cherry Skoal is for somebody who likes the taste of candy, if you know what I'm saying."

In August 2006, U.S. District Court Judge Gladys Kessler released her final opinion in the U.S. Government's landmark case against tobacco companies, meticulously describing how the tobacco companies target youth with sophisticated marketing campaigns. According to Judge Kessler, tobacco companies intimately study youth behavior and use their findings to create images and themes attractive to youth. Judge Kessler found that "defendants spent enormous resources tracking the behaviors and preferences of youth under twenty-one…to start young people smoking and to keep them smoking."

Tobacco companies knowingly placed advertisements in magazines popular with youth, despite the Master Settlement Agreement (MSA), and often sent direct mail pieces to youth without verifying their age.

Judge Kessler's conclusion is very straightforward, "The evidence is clear and convincing—and beyond any reasonable doubt—that defendants have marketed to young people twenty-one and under while consistently, publicly, and falsely denying they do so."

Tobacco Companies Still Market Their Products To Kids

The cigarette companies now claim that they have finally stopped intentionally marketing to kids or targeting youths in their research or promotional efforts. But they continue to advertise cigarettes in ways that reach vulnerable underage populations. For example, the cigarette and spit-tobacco companies continue to advertise heavily at retail outlets near schools and playgrounds, with large ads and signs clearly visible from outside the stores.

Further, a comprehensive report on the media and tobacco use, released by the National Cancer Institute (NCI) in June 2008, describes how tobacco company advertising targets specific population groups, such as youth and young adults, employing themes and messages that resonate with them. For example, tobacco company advertisements suggest that smoking can satisfy adolescents' need to be popular, feel attractive, take risks and avoid or manage stress. In addition:

- A 2008 study of retail outlets in California found that the average number of in-store cigarette ads in California increased between 2002 and 2005, from 22.7 to 24.9 ads per store. The proportion of stores with at least one ad for a sales promotion also increased between 2002 and 2005, from 68.4% to 79.6%.

- A recent survey of 184 retail stores in Hawaii found 3,151 tobacco advertisements and promotions, most of which were for RJ Reynolds' Kool, the cigarette brand most heavily smoked by teenagers in Hawaii.

❖ It's A Fact!!

In fact, cigarette companies increased their spending on point-of-sale marketing by almost $19 million between 2004 and 2005, and spent the bulk of their marketing dollars (81%, or $10.6 billion) on strategies that facilitated retail sales, such as price discounts and ensuring prime retail space.

- A 2002 survey in a Californian community found that stores where adolescents shop most often have more than three times more cigarette advertisements and promotional materials outside of the stores and almost three times more materials inside compared to other stores in the community.

- A 2001 study in the *New England Journal of Medicine* found that the 1998 MSA had little effect on cigarette advertising in magazines. In 2000, the tobacco companies spent $59.6 million in advertising expenditures for the most popular youth brands in youth oriented magazines. The settlement has not reduced youth exposure to advertisements for these brands. Magazine ads for each of the three most popular youth brands (Marlboro, Newport, and Camel) reached more than 80% of young people in the United States an average of 17 times in 2000.

- A Massachusetts Department of Health study found that cigarette advertising in magazines with high youth readership actually increased by 33% after the November 1998 Master Settlement Agreement, in which the tobacco companies agreed not to market to kids. An American Legacy Foundation study found that magazine ads for eight of the top ten cigarette brands reached 70% or more of kids five or more times in 1999.

- In June 2002, a California judge fined the RJ Reynolds cigarette company for advertising in magazines with high youth readerships in ways that violated the state tobacco settlement agreement's prohibition that forbids the cigarette companies from taking any action directly or indirectly to target youth in the advertising, promotion, or marketing of tobacco products.

- In July 2000, a study revealed that after tobacco billboards were banned by the Master Settlement Agreement the cigarette companies increased their advertising and promotions in and around retail outlets, such as convenience stores.

- According to a study conducted by the Massachusetts Department of Health, United States Smokeless Tobacco Company (UST), the country's largest smokeless tobacco manufacturer, spent $9.4 million advertising in magazines with high youth readership in 2001, compared to the average $5.4 million spent in 1997 and 1998, the two years before the settlement. Nearly half of the company's advertising (45%) continued to be in youth-oriented magazines after the settlement.

- At the same time, major cigarette companies vigorously oppose reasonable efforts to make it more difficult for kids to obtain cigarettes—such as raising tobacco excise taxes, eliminating cigarette vending machines in locations accessible by children, requiring that tobacco products be sold from behind the counter, forbidding sales of single cigarettes or "kiddie packs" (packs of fewer than 20 cigarettes), or prohibiting sales of cigarettes via the internet or through the mail. In her final opinion, Judge Kessler noted, "Defendants continue price promotions for premium brands which are most popular with teens."

♣ It's A Fact!!

In fact, the cigarette companies are addicted to underage smoking. Almost 90% of all regular smokers begin smoking at or before age 18, and hardly anybody tries their first cigarette outside of childhood. In other words, if kids stopped smoking, the cigarette companies market of smokers would shrink away to almost nothing. But thanks, in large part, to cigarette company marketing efforts, each day more than 3,500 kids try smoking for the first time, and another 1,000 kids become regular daily smokers.

Empirical Evidence Of The Impact Of Tobacco Marketing To Kids

Beyond the industry's own statements, there is compelling evidence that much of their advertising and promotion is directed at kids and successfully recruits new tobacco users. The 2008 NCI Monograph, noted previously, reflects a comprehensive examination of how mass media is used to encourage and discourage tobacco use. The NCI report found that "the evidence base indicates a causal relationship between tobacco advertising and increased levels of tobacco initiation and continued consumption" and that even brief exposure to tobacco advertising influences adolescents' attitudes and perceptions about smoking as well as their intentions to smoke. The NCI report also found that exposure to depictions of smoking in the movies is causally related to youth smoking initiation.

The 2008 report adds to the findings from an earlier NCI report which reviewed the research on tobacco advertising and promotion and its impact on youth smoking and concluded that there was a causal relationship between tobacco marketing and smoking initiation.

Numerous studies have demonstrated the relationship between tobacco marketing and youth smoking behavior:

- A study published in the May 2007 issue of *Archives of Pediatrics and Adolescent Medicine*, the first national study to examine how specific marketing strategies in convenience stores and other retail settings affect youth smoking, concluded that the more cigarette marketing teens are exposed to in retail stores, the more likely they are to smoke, and that restricting these retail marketing practices would reduce youth smoking. Specifically, the study found that retail cigarette advertising increased the likelihood that youth would initiate smoking; pricing strategies contributed to increases all along the smoking continuum, from initiation and experimentation to regular smoking; and cigarette promotions increased the likelihood that youth will move from experimentation to regular smoking.

- A study published in the December 2006 issue of *Archives of Pediatrics and Adolescent Medicine* found that exposure to tobacco marketing, which includes advertising, promotions and cigarette samples, and to pro-tobacco depictions in films, television, and videos more than doubles the odds that children under 18 will become tobacco users. The researchers also found that pro-tobacco marketing and media depictions lead children who already smoke to smoke more heavily, increasing the odds of progression to heavier use by 42%.

- 81.3% of youth (12–17) smokers prefer Marlboro, Camel and Newport—three heavily advertised brands. Marlboro, the most heavily advertised brand, constitutes almost 50% of the youth market but only about 40% of smokers over age 25.

- A June 2007 study from the American Legacy Foundation found that 40% of youth smokers (ages 13–18) recalled seeing advertisements for flavored cigarettes. Eleven percent of youth smokers have tried flavored cigarettes and more than half of youth smokers who had heard of flavored cigarettes were interested in trying them, with almost 60% believing that flavored cigarettes would taste better than regular cigarettes.

- A study in the *American Journal of Public Health* showed that adolescents who owned a tobacco promotional item and named a cigarette brand whose advertising attracted their attention were twice as likely to become established smokers than those who did neither.

- A survey released in March 2008 showed that kids were almost twice as likely as adults to recall tobacco advertising. While only 24% of all adults recalled seeing a tobacco ad in the two weeks prior to the survey, 47% of kids aged 12 to 17 reported seeing tobacco ads.

- A study in the *Archives of Pediatric and Adolescent Medicine* found that receptivity to tobacco advertising had a significant impact on each step of the progression from nonsmoking to established regular smoking, even when exposure to smoking in the home and by peers was controlled. The biggest impact was on influencing nonsusceptible youth to becoming susceptible to smoking.

- A study in the *Journal of the National Cancer Institute* found that teens are more likely to be influenced to smoke by cigarette advertising than they are by peer pressure.

- A study in the *Journal of Marketing* found that teenagers are three times as sensitive as adults to cigarette advertising.

- A longitudinal study of teenagers in the *Journal of the American Medical Association* showed that tobacco industry promotional activities influenced previously nonsusceptible nonsmokers to become susceptible to or experiment with smoking.

- An *American Journal of Preventive Medicine* study found that youth who were highly receptive to tobacco advertising were 70% more likely to move from being experimental smokers to established smokers compared to those who had a minimal receptivity to tobacco advertising. The study also found that youth who believed that they could quit smoking anytime were almost twice as likely to become established smokers compared to those who did not think they could quit any time.

- According to the U.S. Centers for Disease Control and Prevention, the development and marketing of "starter products" with such features as pouches and cherry flavoring have switched smokeless tobacco from a product used primarily by older men to one used mostly by young men. More than 13% of high school boys are current smokeless tobacco users.

- Between 1989 and 1993, when advertising for the new Joe Camel campaign jumped from $27 million to $43 million, Camel's share among youth increased by more than 50%, while its adult market share did not change at all.

- A report in the *Journal of the American Medical Association* found that six years after the introduction of Virginia Slims and other brands aimed at the female market in the late 1960s, the smoking initiation rate of 12-year-old girls had increased by 110%. Increases among teenage girls of other ages were also substantial.

- A December 1996 survey of advertising industry executives found that roughly 80% believed that advertising for cigarettes reaches children and teenagers in significant numbers and makes smoking more appealing or socially acceptable to kids. And 71% believed that tobacco advertising changes behavior and increases smoking among kids and 59% believe that a goal of tobacco advertising is marketing cigarettes to teenagers who do not already smoke. As a commentator in the Advertising Age trade journal put it, "Cigarette people maintain peer pressure is the culprit in getting kids to start smoking and that advertising has little effect. That's like saying cosmetic ads have no effect on girls too young to put on lipstick."

Chapter 10

The Link Between Youth Smoking And Exposure To Smoking In Movies

Adolescents who see smoking depicted in movies are more likely to become established smokers, according to a study funded by the National Cancer Institute (NCI), part of the National Institutes of Health. The study, which could have broad implications for efforts to reduce smoking among youth, appears in the November 2005 issue of the journal *Pediatrics* and was updated in the September 4, 2007 issue of *Archives of Pediatric Adolescent Medicine*. James Sargent, MD, of Dartmouth-Hitchcock Medical Center in Lebanon, New Hampshire, and colleagues are the first to utilize a nationally representative sample of youth in the United States to examine the influence of adolescents' exposure to movie smoking on their smoking behavior.

Prior research has established that social influences, such as family and peer smoking and tobacco advertising, are important determinants of smoking in adolescents. More recently, research has focused on the impact of smoking in entertainment, including the effect of celebrities who smoke, on youth smoking.

Sargent and his team studied adolescents ages 10 to 14 and found in their earlier study that youth had a higher risk of smoking initiation as their

About This Chapter: From "Increasing Evidence Points to Link Between Youth Smoking and Exposure to Smoking in Movies," National Cancer Institute (www.cancer.gov), September 5, 2007.

exposure to movie smoking increased, with those youth most exposed to movie smoking being most at risk. Adolescents with the greatest exposure to movie smoking were 2.6 times more likely to try smoking than their peers in the least exposed group, after controlling for other factors. The increased risk of smoking initiation associated with exposure to smoking in the movies was similar to that of other well-known risk factors, such as having a parent or sibling who smokes. This increased risk was seen across youth of all racial and ethnic groups, in all geographic regions of the country.

The investigator's latest study examines a more serious behavior outcome: established smoking. Established smokers have smoked more than 100 cigarettes in their lifetimes and most reported symptoms of tobacco addiction and considered themselves smokers. The new study found that teens who had the greatest exposure to smoking in movies were twice as likely to become established smokers, compared with those who had the least exposure. This effect was independent of age, parent, sibling, or friend smoking.

The latest research finding from 2007 also shows that teens who were not sensation-seekers were more responsive to smoking in movies compared with teens who were sensation-seekers. Thus, the effect of movies on behavior may be particularly strong for teens who tend to avoid risk-taking.

"These studies highlight the significant association between smoking in the movies and youth smoking," said Cathy Backinger, PhD, acting chief of NCI's Tobacco Control Research Branch. "These studies reaffirm the need to continue to address the full range of influences on adolescent smoking."

According to the Centers for Disease Control and Prevention, the majority of adult smokers started smoking before the age of 18, and, each day, nearly 4,000 young people try their first cigarette.

"More than 6.4 million children living today will die prematurely because they started smoking as an adolescent," said Backinger. "These statistics demonstrate how crucial it is to address the issue of adolescent smoking."

"Our findings indicate that all U.S. adolescents, regardless of race or place of residence, have a higher risk of trying smoking as their exposure to movie smoking increases," said Sargent. Sargent and his coauthors suggest various approaches to curbing adolescent exposure to movie smoking, including persuading the movie industry to voluntarily reduce depictions of smoking and cigarette brands; incorporating smoking into the movie ratings system to make parents aware of the risks a movie with smoking poses to the adolescent viewer; and encouraging parents to more strongly enforce restrictions on youths' viewing of R-rated movies, which contain the highest amounts of smoking.

"The findings from this national survey complement other studies that showed that exposure to smoking in the movies predicts later youth smoking," said Robert T. Croyle, Ph.D., director of NCI's Division of Cancer Control and Population Sciences. "Now we need to consider effective ways to reduce youths' exposure to this preventable risk factor."

✤ It's A Fact!!

For this research, Sargent and colleagues first analyzed the amount of smoking depicted in the 500 most popular movies released between 1998 and 2002, as well as 32 high-grossing movies released in the first four months of 2003. A "smoking occurrence" was noted when tobacco use was depicted, either by a major or minor character or in the background. By this standard, smoking occurred in 74% of the movies studied. Researchers then conducted a random telephone survey of 6,522 U.S. adolescents ages 10 to 14. Participants were asked whether they had seen a random selection of 50 of the 532 analyzed films. The study participants were also asked, "Have you ever tried smoking a cigarette, even just a puff?" and those who answered "yes" were classified as having tried smoking. The adolescents who participated in the study reported having seen an average of 13 movies, leading to an average exposure to 61 smoking occurrences. Exposure to smoking in movies was significantly higher among Hispanic and black adolescents than among whites.

Chapter 11

Selected Actions Of The U.S. Government Regarding The Regulation Of Tobacco

A Brief Legislative History Of Tobacco Regulation

Pure Food And Drug Act Of 1906

- First federal food and drug law
- No express reference to tobacco products
- Definition of a drug includes medicines and preparations listed in U.S. Pharmacoepia or National Formulary
- 1914 interpretation advised that tobacco be included only when used to cure, mitigate, or prevent disease

Federal Food, Drug, And Cosmetic Act (FFDCA) Of 1938

- Superseded 1906 Act
- Definition of a "drug" includes "articles intended for use in the diagnosis, cure, mitigation, treatment, or prevention of disease in man or other animals" and "articles (other than food) intended to affect the structure or any function of the body of man or other animals"

About This Chapter: This chapter begins with information from "Selected Actions of the U.S. Government Regarding the Regulation of Tobacco Sales, Marketing, and Use (excluding laws pertaining to agriculture or excise tax)," Centers for Disease Control and Prevention (www.cdc.gov), May 29, 2009. Additional information about the Family Smoking Prevention and Tobacco Control Act (2009) is cited separately within the chapter.

- FDA has asserted jurisdiction in cases where the manufacturer or vendor has made medical claims:
    - 1953: Fairfax cigarettes (manufacturer claimed these prevented respiratory and other diseases)
    - 1959: Trim Reducing-Aid Cigarettes (contained the additive tartaric acid, which was claimed to aid in weight reduction)
- FDA has asserted jurisdiction over alternative nicotine-delivery products:
    - 1984: Nicotine Polacrilex gum
    - 1985: Favor Smokeless Cigarette (nicotine-delivery device; ruled a "new drug," intended to treat nicotine dependence and to affect the structure and function of the body; removed from market)
    - 1989: Masterpiece Tobacs tobacco chewing gum; ruled an adulterated food and removed from the market)
    - 1991: Nicotine patches

Federal Trade Commission (FTC) Act Of 1914 (amended in 1938)

- Empowers the FTC to "prevent persons, partnerships, or corporations ... from using unfair or deceptive acts or practices in commerce"

- Between 1945 and 1960, FTC completed seven formal cease-and-desist order proceedings for medical or health claims (for example, a 1942 complaint countering claims that Kool cigarettes provide extra protection against or cure colds)

- In January 1964, FTC proposed a rule to strictly regulate the imagery and copy of cigarette ads to prohibit explicit or implicit health claims

- 1983: FTC determines that its testing procedures may have "significantly underestimated the level of tar, nicotine, and carbon monoxide that smokers received from smoking" certain low-tar cigarettes. Prohibits Brown and Williamson Tobacco Company from using the tar rating for Barclay cigarettes in advertising, packaging, or promotions because of problems with the testing methodology and consumers' possible reliance on that information. FTC authorized revised labeling in 1986.

- 1985: FTC acts to remove the RJ Reynolds advertisements, "Of Cigarettes and Science," in which the multiple risk factor intervention trial (MRFIT) results were misinterpreted

- 1999: FTC requires RJ Reynolds to add a label to packages and ads explaining that "no additives" does not make Winston cigarettes safer

Federal Hazardous Substances Labeling Act (FHSA) Of 1960

- Authorized FDA to regulate substances that are hazardous (either toxic, corrosive, irritant, strong sensitizers, flammable, or pressure-generating). Such substances may cause substantial personal injury or illness during or as a result of customary use.

- 1963: FDA expressed its interpretation that tobacco did not fit the "hazardous" criteria stated previously and withheld recommendations pending the release of the report of the Surgeon General's Advisory Committee on Smoking and Health.

Federal Cigarette Labeling And Advertising Act Of 1965

- Required package warning label—"Caution: Cigarette Smoking May Be Hazardous to Your Health" (other health warnings prohibited)

- Required no labels on cigarette advertisements (in fact, implemented a three-year prohibition of any such labels)

- Required FTC to report to Congress annually on the effectiveness of cigarette labeling, current cigarette advertising and promotion practices, and to make recommendations for legislation

- Required Department of Health, Education, and Welfare (DHEW) to report annually to Congress on the health consequences of smoking

Public Health Cigarette Smoking Act Of 1969

- Required package warning label—"Warning: The Surgeon General Has Determined that Cigarette Smoking Is Dangerous to Your Health" (other health warnings prohibited)

- Temporarily preempted FTC requirement of health labels on advertisements

- Prohibited cigarette advertising on television and radio
- Prevents states or localities from regulating or prohibiting cigarette advertising or promotion for health-related reasons

Controlled Substances Act Of 1970

- To prevent the abuse of drugs, narcotics, and other addictive substances
- Specifically excludes tobacco from the definition of a "controlled substance"

Consumer Product Safety Act Of 1972

- Transferred authority from the FDA to regulate hazardous substances as designated by the Federal Hazardous Substances Labeling Act (FHSA) to the Consumer Product Safety Commission (CPSC)
- The term "consumer product" does not include tobacco and tobacco products

Little Cigar Act Of 1973

- Bans little cigar advertisements from television and radio

1976 Amendment To The Federal Hazardous Substances Labeling Act Of 1960

- The term "hazardous substance" shall not apply to tobacco and tobacco products (passed when the American Public Health Association petitioned CPSC to set a maximum level of 21 mg. of tar in cigarettes)

Toxic Substances Control Act Of 1976

- To "regulate chemical substances and mixtures which present an unreasonable risk of injury to health or the environment"
- The term "chemical substance" does not include tobacco or any tobacco products

Comprehensive Smoking Education Act Of 1984

- Requires four rotating health warning labels (all listed as Surgeon General's Warnings) on cigarette packages and advertisements (smoking causes lung cancer, heart disease and may complicate pregnancy; quitting smoking now greatly reduces serious risks to your health; smoking by pregnant women may result in fetal injury, premature birth, and low birth weight; cigarette smoke contains carbon monoxide) (preempted other package warnings)

- Requires Department of Health and Human Services (DHHS) to publish a biennial status report to Congress on smoking and health

- Creates a Federal Interagency Committee on Smoking and Health

- Requires cigarette industry to provide a confidential list of ingredients added to cigarettes manufactured in or imported into the United States (brand-specific ingredients and quantities not required)

Cigarette Safety Act Of 1984

- To determine the technical and commercial feasibility of developing cigarettes and little cigars that would be less likely to ignite upholstered furniture and mattresses

Comprehensive Smokeless Tobacco Health Education Act Of 1986

- Institutes three rotating health warning labels on smokeless tobacco packages and advertisements (this product may cause mouth cancer; this product may cause gum disease and tooth loss; this product is not a safe alternative to cigarettes) (preempts other health warnings on packages or advertisements [except billboards])

- Prohibits smokeless tobacco advertising on television and radio

- Requires DHHS to publish a biennial status report to Congress on smokeless tobacco

- Requires FTC to report to Congress on smokeless tobacco sales, advertising, and marketing

- Requires smokeless tobacco companies to provide a confidential list of additives and a specification of nicotine content in smokeless tobacco products

- Requires DHHS to conduct public information campaign on the health hazards of smokeless tobacco

Public Law 100-202 (1987)

- Banned smoking on domestic airline flights scheduled for two hours or less

Public Law 101-164 (1989)

- Bans smoking on domestic airline flights scheduled for six hours or less

Synar Amendment To The Alcohol, Drug Abuse, And Mental Health Administration (ADAMHA) Reorganization Act Of 1992

- Requires all states to adopt and enforce restrictions on tobacco sales and distribution to minors

Pro-Children Act Of 1994

- Requires all federally funded children's services to become smoke-free. Expands upon 1993 law that banned smoking in Women, Infants, and Children (WIC) clinics

Family Smoking Prevention And Tobacco Control Act

From "Tobacco Product Labeling and Advertising Warnings," © 2009 Tobacco Control Legal Consortium. All rights reserved. Reprinted with permission. For additional information, visit http://tclconline.org.

Background

On June 22, 2009, President Barack Obama signed into law the Family Smoking Prevention and Tobacco Control Act, giving the U.S. Food and Drug Administration (FDA) comprehensive authority to regulate the manufacturing, marketing, and sale of tobacco products. The new law represents the most sweeping action taken to date to reduce what remains the leading preventable cause of death in the United States.

Before now, tobacco products were largely exempt from regulation under the nation's federal health and safety laws, including the Food, Drug, and Cosmetic Act. The FDA has regulated food, drugs, and cosmetics for many decades, but not tobacco products, except in those rare circumstances when manufacturers made explicit health claims.

✤ It's A Fact!!
What are some of the key regulatory timelines associated with the FSPTCA?

There are many requirements with deadlines outlined in the Family Smoking Prevention and Tobacco Control Act (FSPTCA). Some highlights include the following:

- By October 2009, cigarettes will be prohibited from having candy, fruit, and spice flavors as their characterizing flavors.

- By January 2010, tobacco manufacturers and importers will submit information to the U.S. Food and Drug Administration (FDA) about ingredients and additives in tobacco products.

- By April 2010, FDA will reissue the 1996 regulation aimed at reducing young people's access to tobacco products and curbing the appeal of tobacco to the young.

- By July 2010, tobacco manufacturers may no longer use the terms "light," "low," and "mild" on tobacco products without an FDA order in effect.

- By July 2010, warning labels for smokeless tobacco products will be revised and strengthened.

- By October 2012, warning labels for cigarettes will be revised and strengthened.

Source: Excerpted from "Frequently Asked Questions on the Passage of the Family Smoking Prevention and Tobacco Control Act (FSPTCA)," U.S. Food and Drug Administration, 2009.

What The New Law Does

The new law prescribes stronger health warning labels on tobacco product packages and advertisements. Currently, the warning labels for cigarettes read as follows, as they have for the past quarter century:

- SURGEON GENERAL'S WARNING: Smoking Causes Lung Cancer, Heart Disease, Emphysema, and May Complicate Pregnancy

- SURGEON GENERAL'S WARNING: Quitting Smoking Now Greatly Reduces Serious Risks to Your Health

- SURGEON GENERAL'S WARNING: Smoking by Pregnant Women May Result in Fetal Injury, Premature Birth, and Low Birth Weight

- SURGEON GENERAL'S WARNING: Cigarette Smoke Contains Carbon Monoxide

Under the new law, the warnings for cigarettes will be changed to read as follows (no later than 39 months after enactment):

- WARNING: Cigarettes are addictive

- WARNING: Tobacco smoke can harm your children

- WARNING: Cigarettes cause fatal lung disease

♣ It's A Fact!!
Flavored Tobacco

On September 22, 2009 a ban on cigarettes containing certain characterizing flavors went into effect. The ban, authorized by the new Family Smoking Prevention and Tobacco Control Act, is part of a national effort by the U.S. Food and Drug Administration (FDA) to reduce smoking in America.

FDA's ban on candy and fruit-flavored cigarettes highlights the importance of reducing the number of children who start to smoke, and who become addicted to dangerous tobacco products. FDA is also examining options for regulating both menthol cigarettes and flavored tobacco products other than cigarettes.

According to the act:

> …a cigarette or any of its component parts (including the tobacco, filter, or paper) shall not contain, as a constituent (including a smoke constituent) or additive, an artificial or natural flavor (other than tobacco or menthol) or an herb or spice, including strawberry, grape, orange, clove, cinnamon, pineapple, vanilla, coconut, licorice, cocoa, chocolate, cherry, or coffee, that is a characterizing flavor of the tobacco product or tobacco smoke

Any company who continues to make, ship or sell such products may be subject to FDA enforcement actions. You are encouraged to report any company that sells cigarettes with these certain characterizing flavors.

Source: From "Tobacco Products: Flavored Tobacco," U.S. Food and Drug Administration (FDA), 2009.

- WARNING: Cigarettes cause cancer

- WARNING: Cigarettes cause strokes and heart disease

- WARNING: Smoking during pregnancy can harm your baby

- WARNING: Smoking can kill you

- WARNING: Tobacco smoke causes fatal lung disease in nonsmokers

- WARNING: Quitting smoking now greatly reduces serious risks to your health

The law mandates that the new warnings cover 50% of the top half of the front and back of each pack with graphics depicting the health consequences of tobacco use, and that the word "WARNING" appear in 7-point type in black and white text only. Warnings will be randomly displayed in each two-month period and rotated quarterly.

Currently, the warning labels for smokeless tobacco products read as follows:

- WARNING: This product may cause mouth cancer

- WARNING: This product may cause gum disease and tooth loss

- WARNING: This product is not a safe alternative to cigarettes

Under the legislation, the warnings for smokeless tobacco products will be changed to read as follows (two months after enactment):

- WARNING: This product can cause mouth cancer

- WARNING: This product can cause gum disease and tooth loss

- WARNING: This product is not a safe alternative to cigarettes

- WARNING: Smokeless tobacco is addictive

The smokeless tobacco warnings will cover 30% of the two principal display panels of each package, and the word "WARNING" will appear in 7-point type in black and white text only. Warnings will be randomly displayed in each two-month period and rotated quarterly.

The law requires the placement of the same cigarette and smokeless to-bacco product warning labels in advertisements, rotated at random and in equal proportion in each two-month period. The warnings will comprise at least 20% of the entire area of each advertisement and appear in black and white text only.

The FDA is also authorized to further revise the labeling requirements for cigarettes and smokeless tobacco products, including changing the text, format and type size, without new action by Congress. The FDA may also establish warning labels on other tobacco products.

Through an amendment to the Federal Cigarette Labeling and Advertising Act, the new law grants the FDA authority to require the posting of information concerning tar and nicotine yields on cigarette packages or advertisements. The FDA can also require disclosure of information relating to other tobacco product constituents—in package or advertising inserts, or in other ways—if the agency determines that such disclosure would benefit public health or otherwise increase consumer awareness of the health consequences of tobacco use.

Unrelated to warning labels per se, but likewise affecting the messages to which consumers are exposed, the law prohibits the use of such terms as "light," "mild" and "low-tar" on tobacco product packages and in advertisements because of such terms mislead consumers into believing that certain cigarettes are safer than others.

To learn more about FDA regulation of tobacco, visit www.tclconline.org.

Part Two

Nicotine Delivery Systems

Chapter 12

Cigarettes And Brand Preferences

The National Survey on Drug Use and Health (NSDUH) asked people aged 12 or older to report whether they smoked part or all of a cigarette in the past 30 days. Respondents who reported smoking part or all of a cigarette in the past 30 days were asked to report which cigarette brand they smoked most often during that time. This chapter presents data on the prevalence of cigarette smoking in the past month among the U.S. civilian, noninstitutionalized population aged 12 or older, as well as information on cigarette brand preferences.

Cigarette Prevalence

According to the 2005 NSDUH, 24.9% of persons aged 12 or older (60.5 million persons) smoked part or all of a cigarette during the past month. In the past month, 10.8% of youths aged 12 to 17, 39.0% of young adults aged 18 to 25, and 24.3% of adults 26 or older smoked cigarettes, as did about one quarter of males (27.4%) and females (22.5%).

Among whites, 26.0% were past month cigarette smokers, as were 24.5% of blacks and 22.1% of Hispanics. Cigarette smoking in the past month was reported by 28.1% of persons aged 12 or older who were living in the Midwest, 25.6% of those living in the South, 24.5% of those living in the Northeast, and 21.0% of those living in the West.

About This Chapter: Text in this chapter is from "Cigarette Brand Preferences in 2005," *The NSDUH Report*, Substance Abuse and Mental Health Services Administration, January 2007.

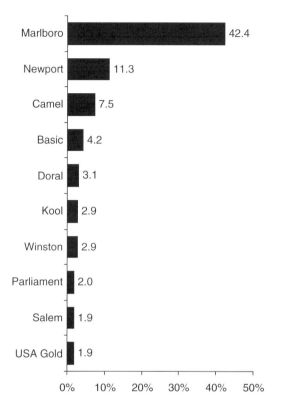

Figure 12.1. *Percentages of Past Month Cigarette Smokers Aged 12 or Older Reporting Cigarette Brands Used Most Often During the Past Month: 2005 (Source: SAMHSA, 2005 NSDUH).*

Cigarette Brands Used Most Often

In 2005, Marlboro was the brand used most often by past month cigarette smokers, followed by Newport, Camel, Basic, and Doral. The remainder of the 10 brands used most often included Kool, Winston, Parliament, Salem, and USA Gold.

Demographic Differences In Cigarette Brand Use

Research has shown that cigarette brand use varies by age, gender, and race/ethnicity. Among past month smokers in 2005, Marlboro was the brand used most often in the past month by youths aged 12 to 17 (48.0%), young adults aged 18 to 25 (50.8%), and older adults aged 26 or older (39.8%)

✎ What's It Mean?

<u>Cigarette:</u> The Federal Cigarette Labeling and Advertising Act (FCLAA), 15 U.S.C. §1332(1)(A) and (B) defines a cigarette as "any roll of tobacco wrapped in paper or in any substance not containing tobacco…[and] any roll of tobacco wrapped in any substance containing tobacco which, because of its appearance, the type of tobacco used in the filler, or its packaging and labeling, is likely to be offered to, or purchased by, consumers as a cigarette…"

Source: Excerpted from "Key Terms and Definitions," Centers for Disease Control and Prevention, May 29, 2009.

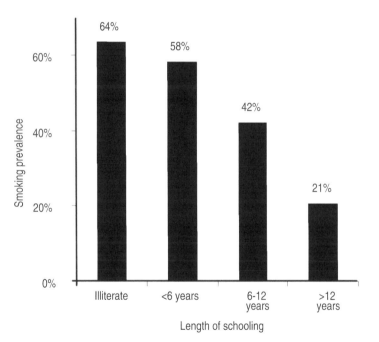

Source: Gajalakshmi, C. K., P. Jha, S. Nguyen, and A. Yurekli. *Patterns of Tobacco Use, and Health Consequences.* Background paper.

Figure 12.2. *Percentages of Past Month Cigarette Smokers Aged 12 or Older Reporting Cigarette Brands Used Most Often During the Past Month, by Age group: 2005 (Source: SAMHSA, 2005 NSDUH).*

Adults aged 26 or older reported a somewhat greater diversity of brand preference compared with youths and young adults. The five brands used most often by youths and young adults accounted for 86.0% of youths and 89.2% of young adults who smoked cigarettes in the past month. Nevertheless, the five brands used most among smokers aged 26 or older still accounted for 63.2% of smokers in this age group.

Among whites who smoked cigarettes in the past month, Marlboro was the brand used most often in the past month, followed by Camel. Marlboro was also the brand used most often by Hispanics, followed by Newport. Among blacks, Newport was the brand used most often, followed by Kool, both of which are menthol cigarettes.

✤ It's A Fact!!
Does the filter on your cigarette really make it safer?

Most people mistakenly believe that smoking a filtered cigarette is safer than smoking an nonfiltered cigarette. This is false.

Health studies show that smoking filtered cigarettes do not keep you from getting sick. Filters do not protect you from bad chemicals and, in some ways, they may be more dangerous than nonfiltered cigarettes.

Why don't filters work?

- Filters do not block all the bad chemicals in smoke.
- Filtered smoke feels milder on the throat, making it easier to take bigger and deeper puffs.
- Filters help block only the biggest tar particles while letting through the smaller bits of tar that can travel deeper into your lungs.

Filters are defective—and the companies know it. You may be inhaling filter fibers into your lungs.

- Most cigarette filters are made of the same material as camera film (cellulose acetate).
- Each individual filter is made of thousands of tiny fibers.
- The inside of the filter is painted white to make it appear clean.

Among persons aged 12 or older who smoked cigarettes in the past month, males (44.6%) and females (40.0%) were more likely to smoke Marlboro than any other brand. Newport was the second-most used brand among males and females (10.8 and 11.8%, respectively), and Camel ranked third (9.7 and 5.0%, respectively).

Geographic Differences In Cigarette Brand Use

Marlboro was the cigarette brand used most often by past month cigarette smokers in all four geographic regions. Newport was second in prevalence in the Northeast, Midwest, and South, while Camel was second in the West.

- During smoking, these fibers can come off into your mouth and be inhaled into your lungs.

Charcoal filters are no better. If you smoke a cigarette with a charcoal filter, not only can you get fibers in your body, you can also get tiny bits of charcoal.

What cigarette manufacturers will not tell you:

- Tobacco industry documents show that they have known about filter fiber fallout since at least the 1950s:

  > "Carbon particles were released from all cigarettes tested. In some studies, the particles released from cigarette filters were described as: "..too numerous to count." —Memo to Judy Nash from Nancy R. Ryan. February 18, 1982. "Filter particle fallout." Bates No. 1000805035.

  > "He said when [a filter] plug is cut ...there always remains a few loose, hard particles of filament. These loose, hard pieces of material are then sucked down into the lungs of the smoker." —Memo to Mr. O.P. McComas from Anne C. Stubing. May 1, 1957. (no title). Bates No. 2040015018-2040015020.

Don't be fooled: The filter on your cigarette may be causing you more harm than good.

Source: "Your Cigarettes May Be Killing You," © New York State Smokers' Quitline (www.nysmokefree.com). Reprinted with permission.

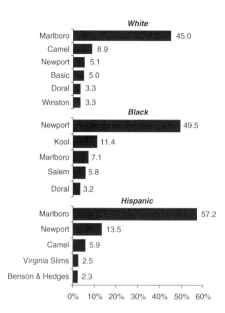

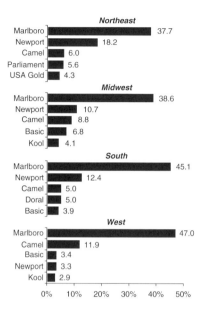

Figure 12.3. *Percentages of Past Month Cigarette Smokers Aged 12 or Older Reporting Cigarette Brands Used Most Often During the Past Month, by Race/ Ethnicity*: 2005 (Source: SAMHSA, 2005 NSDUH).*

Figure 12.4. *Percentages of Past Month Cigarette Smokers Aged 12 or Older Reporting Cigarette Brands Used Most Often During the Past Month, by Region: 2005 (Source: SAMHSA, 2005 NSDUH).*

Marlboro was the cigarette brand used most often by past month cigarette smokers in large metropolitan, small metropolitan, and non-metropolitan areas (43.6, 41.6, and 40.5%, respectively). Newport was the second-most prevalent brand in large metropolitan (14.0%) and small metropolitan (10.0%) areas, while Camel was the second-most prevalent brand in non-metropolitan areas (7.4%).

Chapter 13

"Light" Cigarettes

Many smokers choose "low-tar," "mild," "light," or "ultra-light" cigarettes because they think that these cigarettes may be less harmful to their health than "regular" or "full-flavor" cigarettes. Although smoke from light cigarettes may feel smoother and lighter on the throat and chest, light cigarettes are not healthier than regular cigarettes. The truth is that light cigarettes do not reduce the health risks of smoking. The only way to reduce a smoker's risk, and the risk to others, is to stop smoking completely.

What about the lower tar and nicotine numbers on light and ultra-light cigarette packs and in ads for these products?

These numbers come from smoking machines, which "smoke" every brand of cigarettes exactly the same way.

These numbers do not really tell how much tar and nicotine a particular smoker may get because people do not smoke cigarettes the same way the machines do. And no two people smoke the same way.

How do light cigarettes trick the smoking machines?

Tobacco companies designed light cigarettes with tiny pinholes on the filters. These "filter vents" dilute cigarette smoke with air when light cigarettes

About This Chapter: Text in this chapter is from "The Truth about 'Light' Cigarettes: Questions and Answers," National Cancer Institute, August 17, 2004.

are "puffed" on by smoking machines, causing the machines to measure artificially low tar and nicotine levels.

Many smokers do not know that their cigarette filters have vent holes. The filter vents are uncovered when cigarettes are smoked on smoking machines. However, filter vents are placed just millimeters from where smokers put their lips or fingers when smoking. As a result, many smokers block the vents—which actually turns the light cigarette into a regular cigarette.

Some cigarette makers increased the length of the paper wrap covering the outside of the cigarette filter, which decreases the number of puffs that occur during the machine test. Although tobacco under the wrap is still available to the smoker, this tobacco is not burned during the machine test. The result is that the machine measures less tar and nicotine levels than is available to the smoker.

Because smokers, unlike machines, crave nicotine, they may inhale more deeply; take larger, more rapid, or more frequent puffs; or smoke a few extra cigarettes each day to get enough nicotine to satisfy their craving. This is called "compensating," and it means that smokers end up inhaling more tar, nicotine, and other harmful chemicals than the machine-based numbers suggest.

✤ It's A Fact!!

You may think that "light" cigarettes aren't as bad as regular cigarettes. Think again. Light cigarettes put smokers at the same risk for smoking-related health problems as regular cigarettes.

Some cigarette packs say that light cigarettes have lower tar and nicotine. Don't let these claims fool you. Tobacco companies use smoking machines to figure out the amount of tar and nicotine in the cigarettes. These machines "smoke" every brand of cigarettes the same way. However, people don't smoke cigarettes the same way machines do. People who smoke light cigarettes may inhale more deeply, take more puffs, or smoke extra cigarettes to satisfy their nicotine craving. As a result, they may inhale just as much tar, nicotine, and other chemicals as people who smoke regular cigarettes.

Source: From "Smoking and How to Quit: 'Light' Cigarettes," National Women's Health Information Center (www.womenshealth.gov), June 17, 2009.

What is the scientific evidence about the health effects of light cigarettes?

The federal government's National Cancer Institute has concluded that light cigarettes provide no benefit to smokers' health.

According to the National Cancer Institute monograph *Risks Associated with Smoking Cigarettes with Low Machine-Measured Yields of Tar and Nicotine*, people who switch to light cigarettes from regular cigarettes are likely to inhale the same amount of hazardous chemicals, and they remain at high risk for developing smoking-related cancers and other diseases.

Researchers also found that the strategies used by the tobacco industry to advertise and promote light cigarettes are intended to reassure smokers, to discourage them from quitting, and to lead consumers to perceive filtered and light cigarettes as safer alternatives to regular cigarettes.

There is also no evidence that switching to light or ultra-light cigarettes actually helps smokers quit.

Have the tobacco companies conducted research on the amount of tar and nicotine people actually inhale while smoking light cigarettes?

The tobacco industry's own documents show that companies are aware that smokers of light cigarettes compensate by taking bigger puffs.

Industry documents also show that the companies are aware of the difference between machine-measured yields of tar and nicotine and what the smoker actually inhales.

What is the bottom line for smokers who want to protect their health?

There is no such thing as a safe cigarette. The only proven way to reduce the risk of smoking-related disease is to quit smoking completely.

Smokers who quit live longer than those who continue to smoke. In addition, the earlier smokers quit, the greater the health benefit. Research has shown that people who quit before age 30 eliminate almost all of their risk of developing a tobacco-related disease. Even smokers who quit at age 50 reduce their risk of dying from a tobacco-related disease.

Quitting also decreases the risk of lung cancer, heart attacks, stroke, and chronic lung disease.

Chapter 14

Menthol Cigarettes

Introduction

Menthol is unique in that it is the only cigarette additive that is actively marketed to consumers. It is the only aspect of cigarette design that is explicitly marketed based on its physiological effects, as an anti-irritant and a cooling agent. It is the only cigarette additive about which consumers make conscious buying choices.

The Emergence Of Menthol Cigarettes

Menthol cigarettes were conceived as specialty products in the 1920s and 1930s. These cigarettes were initially marketed as a luxury product, through radio and magazine ads, and especially targeted to women smokers. Until the 1960s, the market share of menthol cigarettes never exceeded 5%. However, with the great migration of African Americans from the South to urban centers, peaking during and after World War II, the industry started targeting menthol cigarettes to African Americans. Launched in the early 1940s, the popular African American magazines (for example, *Ebony*, *Jet*) offered a

About This Chapter: This chapter begins with an excerpt from "The First Conference on Menthol Cigarettes: Setting the Research Agenda, Executive Summary," U.S. Department of Health and Human Services, 2003. "Use of Menthol Cigarettes," is from *The NSDUH Report*, National Survey on Drug Use and Health, Substance Abuse and Mental Health Services Administration, November 29, 2009.

unique opportunity for precision marketing. By the 1960s and 1970s, menthol brands had become the cigarettes of choice for the majority of African American smokers. Whereas only about 25% of white smokers use menthol cigarettes, more than 70% of African American smokers choose them; other population segments are now adopting menthol use, including young people, Asian and Pacific Islander Americans, and women.

Today, menthol cigarettes represent about 26% of all cigarettes sold in the United States. Newport cigarettes are the leading menthol brand and are second only to Marlboro in overall market share.

The Importance Of Studying Menthol Cigarettes

One urgent question that needs to be answered is whether menthol cigarettes contribute to the health disparities between white and African American smokers. Although African Americans tend to smoke fewer cigarettes per day than do white smokers, incidence and mortality rates of lung cancer and mortality rates of lung cancer and other smoking-related diseases are significantly higher among African Americans. Historically, the age-adjusted smoking-related lung cancer death rates in the United States among African American males and white males were: in 1950, 15.7 and 21.9, respectively; in 1965, 47.8 and 47.3, respectively; and in 1990, 107.7 and 73.6, respectively. Whether these trends reflect the trends of use of menthol cigarettes by African Americans remains to be determined.

Menthol, a chemical compound extracted from the peppermint plant and classified as a mild local anesthetic, was commonly used in veterinary medicine. Colorless and with a mint scent, menthol was first added to cigarettes in the 1920s and 1930s to mask the harshness of tobacco smoke. Fifty-two percent of 174 African Americans interviewed in one study reported that mentholated cigarettes were less harsh on the throat, 48% stated that inhalation was easier, and 33% felt they could inhale more deeply.

Since the 1960s, menthol brands have been marketed by the industry as "refreshing" and "cool." Menthol stimulates cold receptors, with the resulting sensation of coolness perceived not only in the mouth and pharynx, but also in the lungs. Stimulation of laryngeal cold receptors may reduce airway irritation.

This sensation of coolness might result in deeper inhalation, but because of the difficulty in precisely measuring the inhalation phase of smoking, this issue has not been adequately studied. Menthol may increase salivary flow thereby enhancing the passage of harmful smoke constituents across mucus membranes.

Menthol has been shown to increase significantly involuntary breath holding. Breath holding at peak inspiration could contribute to increased uptake of inhaled tobacco smoke constituents, including nicotine and cancer-causing agents, from the alveoli of the lungs into the bloodstream.

There have been conflicting reports on the effect of menthol on smoking topography (for example, puff volume, puff frequency) that may be due to small samples and variations in study populations. The 1999 Massachusetts Benchmark Study of the 24 most popular U.S. filter cigarette brands and styles (six of them were menthol brands) provided some evidence that the chemical composition of the mainstream smoke of selected menthol cigarettes differs from that of their nonmenthol counterparts.

The yields of "tar," nicotine, carbon monoxide, and several carcinogenic compounds (for example, benzene, 1,3-butadiene, benzo[a]pyrene, NNK), obtained by the Massachusetts machine-smoking method, were 30–70% higher in the mainstream smoke of menthol cigarettes than in the smoke of the selected nonmentholated brands. There are many cigarette design characteristics (for example, tobacco blend, resistance to draw, paper porosity, amount of tobacco in the rod, cigarette length, and others) that may contribute to differences in yield that are independent of mentholation.

❖ It's A Fact!!

Menthol cigarettes have a minty taste that makes some smokers think they are healthier than regular cigarettes. This is not true! In fact, menthol cigarettes contain even more chemicals than regular cigarettes. Also, menthol can make it easier for a smoker to inhale deeply, which may allow more chemicals to enter the lungs. As a result, menthol cigarettes may be even more harmful than regular cigarettes.

Source: Excerpted from "Smoking and How to Quit," National Women's Health Information Center (www.womenshealth.gov), June 17, 2009.

For example, Newport, the most popular menthol brand in the United States, is a "full flavor" cigarette with no filter ventilation holes, while the most popular nonmentholated brand, "full flavor" Marlboro, averages 8% ventilation in the hard pack version and 11% ventilation in the soft pack.

❖ It's A Fact!!

Most African American smokers smoke menthols. As smoking rates have gone down among whites, cigarette companies have worked hard to hook more African Americans on menthol cigarettes. For example, the company that makes Kool cigarettes recently launched an ad campaign featuring young hip hop artists in hopes of getting more young African Americans hooked on their cigarettes.

Source: Excerpted from "Smoking and How to Quit," National Women's Health Information Center (www.womenshealth.gov), June 17, 2009.

Use Of Menthol Cigarettes

The National Survey on Drug Use and Health (NSDUH) asks persons aged 12 or older about whether or not they smoked part or all of a cigarette in the past 30 days. Respondents who answered affirmatively are asked whether or not the cigarettes they smoked during the past 30 days were menthol and how many days they smoked during the past month. Additionally, persons who had ever smoked a cigarette are asked how old they were when they first began smoking cigarettes; responses are used to identify recent initiates (that is, persons who used cigarettes for the first time in the 12 months prior to the survey).

This text examines the prevalence of use of menthol cigarettes among past month smokers. The first section presents data on trends in use between 2004 and 2008. Findings in the remainder of the report are annual averages based on combined 2004 to 2008 NSDUH data.

Trends In Menthol Cigarette Use Among Past Month Smokers

Overall, the rate of smoking menthol cigarettes among past month smokers increased from 31.0% in 2004 to 33.9% in 2008. Rates of menthol use increased from 43.5 to 47.7% among adolescents aged 12 to 17 and from 34.1

Table 14.1. Trends in past month menthol cigarette use among past month cigarette smokers aged 12 or older, by age group—2004 to 2008

Age Group	2004	2005	2006	2007	2008
Aged 12 to 17	43.5%	41.5%	44.5%	47.7%	47.7%
Aged 18 to 25	34.1%	34.0%	35.6%	38.5%	40.8%
Aged 26 or Older	29.3%	29.4%	29.9%	30.4%	31.5%

Source: 2004 to 2008 SAMHSA National Surveys on Drug Use and Health (NSDUHs).

Table 14.2. Trends in past month menthol cigarette use among past month cigarette smokers aged 12 or older, by gender—2004 to 2008

Gender	2004	2005	2006	2007	2008
Male	26.9%	26.5%	28.1%	29.2%	30.8%
Female	35.9%	36.0%	35.8%	36.7%	37.5%

Source: 2004 to 2008 SAMHSA National Surveys on Drug Use and Health (NSDUHs).

to 40.8% among young adults aged 18 to 25. Rates also generally increased among males, from 26.9 to 30.8%.

Use Of Menthol Cigarettes Among Past Month Smokers

Combined 2004 to 2008 data indicate that nearly one third (32.0%) of past month smokers aged 12 or older smoked menthol cigarettes in the past month. The prevalence of menthol cigarette use among past month smokers decreased with age (44.8% among smokers aged 12 to 17, 36.5% among those aged 18 to 25, and 30.1% among those aged 26 or older), and it was more likely among females than males (36.4 vs. 28.3%). Rates of menthol cigarette use varied greatly by race/ethnicity, ranging from 82.6% among blacks to 23.8% among whites.

Over three fifths of past month smokers (62.1%) smoked daily, and they were less likely than less frequent smokers to have used menthol cigarettes in the past month (30.1 vs. 35.1%).

Table 14.3. Past month menthol cigarette use among past month cigarette smokers aged 12 or older, by age group and gender—2004 to 2008

Age Group	Percent
Aged 12 to 17	44.8%
Aged 18 to 25	36.5%
Aged 26 or Older	30.1%

Gender	
Male	28.3%
Female	36.4%

Source: 2004 to 2008 SAMHSA National Surveys on Drug Use and Health (NSDUHs).

✤ **It's A Fact!!**

Since the 1964 publication of the first Surgeon General's Report on Smoking, the Nation's level of awareness on the adverse health consequences of cigarettes has steadily increased. Federal, state, and local laws have increasingly restricted sales of tobacco products, raised taxes on these products, and curtailed the venues in which these products can be used. The data from NSDUH point out, however, that the initiation of tobacco products—particularly cigarettes—continues to be a public health problem. This appears to be especially true for menthol cigarettes and adolescents. Although research continues into the effects of menthol, prevention specialists may wish to consider prevention strategies for adolescents that are more targeted at the initiation of menthol cigarette use and the attractions of a "cooler" taste. Similarly, professionals involved in smoking cessation programs may want to consider whether or not menthol cigarette smokers need different or ancillary strategies and supports to become smoke-free.

Source: Substance Abuse and Mental Health Services Administration, November 29, 2009.

Table 14.4. Past month menthol cigarette use among past month cigarette smokers aged 12 or older, by race/ethnicity—2004 to 2008

Race/Ethnicity	Percent
Black or African American	82.6%
Native Hawaiian or Other Pacific Islander	53.2%
Two or More Races	36.9%
Hispanic or Latino	32.3%
Asian	31.2%
American Indian or Alaska Native	24.8%
White	23.8%

Source: 2004 to 2008 SAMHSA National Surveys on Drug Use and Health (NSDUHs).

Table 14.5. Past month menthol cigarette use among past month cigarette smokers aged 12 or older, by recency of cigarette initiation and demographic characteristics: 2004 to 2008

Demographic Characteristic	Past Year Initiate	Initiated Use More Than One Year Ago
Total		
Aged 12 or Older	44.6%	31.8%
Age Group*		
Aged 12 to 17	49.2%	43.8%
Aged 18 to 25	40.2%	36.4%
Gender		
Male	42.6%	28.1%
Female	46.6%	36.2%
Race/Ethnicity*		
Black	73.9%	82.8%
Hispanic	42.9%	32.1%
White	39.9%	23.6%

* Data for those aged 26 or older and for other racial/ethnic groups are not presented because of low precision.

Source: 2004 to 2008 SAMHSA National Surveys on Drug Use and Health (NSDUHs).

Use Of Menthol Cigarettes, By Recency Of Cigarette Initiation

Most past month smokers (98.3%) initiated cigarette smoking more than 12 months before the survey (that is, were longer term smokers). Past month use of menthol cigarettes was more likely among smokers who started in the past 12 months than among longer term smokers (44.6 vs. 31.8%). This pattern was consistent for persons aged 12 to 17 and those aged 18 to 25, for both genders, and for whites and Hispanics.

For blacks, however, this pattern was reversed. Past month use of menthol cigarettes was less likely among recent smoking initiates than among longer term smokers (73.9 vs. 82.8%). Blacks who were recent initiates of cigarette smoking were about 1.9 times more likely than whites to have used menthol cigarettes in the past month; in comparison, blacks who were longer term smokers were 3.5 times more likely than whites to have done so.

Chapter 15

Electronic Cigarettes

Electronic Cigarette ("E-Cigarette") Fact Sheet

Electronic cigarettes ("e-cigarettes") are devices, about the size of a regular cigarette. They operate by electronically vaporizing a solution that often contains nicotine, creating a mist which is then inhaled. E-cigarettes are available in various flavors and claimed strengths of nicotine cartridges.

How An Electronic Cigarette Works

- When a user inhales on the mouthpiece, the vaporizer is turned on and converts the liquid in the cartridge into a vapor. A rechargeable battery powers the vaporizer and has an indicator light to show when the device is in use.[1]

- The components of a typical e-cigarette are the mouthpiece, cartridge, vaporizer, battery, and indicator light.

- Cartridges generally contain nicotine, flavoring, and other chemicals.[2] Quality control of the ingredients is of concern.[3] For more details, see the section below, "Safety and Quality Control."

- Cartridges are sold with various amounts of nicotine, from 0 mg to 18 mg of nicotine or more, although the U.S. Food and Drug Administration (FDA) testing has shown that these advertised strengths can be very different than the actual amount of nicotine in the cartridges.[2]

- Some users refill their own cartridges, which may be dangerous because it involves dealing with toxic levels of nicotine. Some refill bottles contain over 1,000 mg of nicotine, and the fatal dose for children is estimated at only 10 mg and for adults is estimated at 30–60 mg.[4]

Manufacturers

- Ruyan, a Chinese company, claims to have originally invented and patented the e-cigarette.[5]

> ### ✎ What's It Mean?
>
> Electronic Cigarettes: Also known as "e-cigarettes," electronic cigarettes are battery-operated devices designed to look like and to be used in the same manner as conventional cigarettes. Sold online and in many shopping malls, the devices generally contain cartridges filled with nicotine, flavor, and other chemicals. They turn nicotine, which is highly addictive, and other chemicals into a vapor that is inhaled by the user.
>
> Source: "FDA Warns of Health Risks Posed by E-Cigarettes," U.S. Food and Drug Administration (www.fda.gov), July 23, 2009.

- There are now a number of companies selling e-cigarettes both on the internet and in retail mall locations in the U.S., including Ruyan, Crown 7, ePuffer, Gamucci, Janty, NJOY, PureSmoker, S.S. Choice, SmokeStik, and Smoking Everywhere.

Legal Status

- The FDA has classified the e-cigarettes it has examined as combination drug-device products that would require FDA approval before being legally sold in the U.S.[6]

- The FDA has been challenged regarding its jurisdiction over e-cigarettes in a case currently pending in federal district court (Smoking Everywhere v. FDA No. 1:09-CV-0077-RJL (D.D.C.).[6]

- Internationally, the legality of e-cigarettes varies; for example, they are banned in Canada and Australia.[7,8]

Potential Youth Appeal

- There is concern that electronic cigarettes may appeal to youth because of their high-tech design, easy availability online or via mall kiosks, and the wide array of flavors of cartridges including chocolate and mint.[6]

Safety And Quality Control

While some manufacturers have funded research on electronic cigarettes, at this point the only independent research on e-cigarettes available has been done by the FDA and was released on July 22, 2009.[1]

The FDA's Division of Pharmaceutical Analysis analyzed the ingredients in a small sample of cartridges from two leading brands of electronic cigarettes, and found that the tested products contained detectable levels of known carcinogens (chemicals that cause cancer) and toxic chemicals.[3] In one sample, the FDA detected diethylene glycol, a chemical used in antifreeze that is toxic to humans.[3] In several other samples, the FDA detected carcinogens, including nitrosamines.[3]

The FDA's other important findings include the following:

• The testing suggested that the quality control processes used to manufacture these products are inconsistent or non-existent.[3] For example, three different e-cigarette cartridges with the same label were tested and each cartridge emitted a markedly different amount of nicotine with each puff.

• The e-cigarette cartridges that were labeled as containing no nicotine had low levels of nicotine in all cartridges tested, except one.[3]

❖ It's A Fact!!

The U.S. Food and Drug Administration warns consumers about potential health risks associated with electronic cigarettes. The FDA's concerns include the following:

• E-cigarettes can increase nicotine addiction among young people and may lead kids to try other tobacco products, including conventional cigarettes, which are known to cause disease and lead to premature death.

• The products may contain ingredients that are known to be toxic to humans.

• Because clinical studies about the safety and efficacy of these products for their intended use have not been submitted to FDA, consumers currently have no way of knowing whether e-cigarettes are safe for their intended use, or about what types or concentrations of potentially harmful chemicals or what dose of nicotine they are inhaling when they use these products.

- In addition to the known carcinogens and toxic chemicals, tobacco-specific impurities suspected of being harmful to humans, anabasine, myosmine, and β-nicotyrine, were detected in a majority of the samples tested.[3]

- One high-nicotine cartridge delivered twice as much nicotine to users when the vapor from that e-cigarette brand was inhaled than was delivered by a sample of the nicotine inhalation product approved by the FDA for use as a smoking cessation aid that was used as a control.[3]

Sources

1. Westenberger, B.J., Evaluation of e-cigarettes. 2009, FDA, Center for Drug Evaluation and Research, Division of Pharmaceutical Analysis: St. Louis, MO.

2. FDA. *Consumer Updates: FDA Warns of Health Risks Posed by E-Cigarettes.* 2009 July 24, 2009 [cited 2009 August 12, 2009]; Available from: http://www.fda.gov/ForConsumers/ConsumerUpdates/ucm173401.htm.

3. FDA. *Summary of results: Laboratory analysis of electronic cigarettes conducted by FDA.* 2009 July 22, 2009 [cited 2009 August 12, 2009]; Available from: http://www.fda.gov/NewsEvents/PublicHealthFocus/ucm173146.htm.

4. INCHEM, I.P.o.C.S.I. *Nicotine.* 1991 [cited 2009 August 12, 2009]; Available from: http://www.inchem.org/documents/pims/chemical/nicotine.htm.

5. Ruyan. *Ruyan asserts patent rights to e-cigarette in key China court ruling.* 2009 [cited 2009 August 12, 2009]; Available from: http://www.ruyanamerica.com/News/News.cfm?NewsID=1008.

6. FDA. FDA and public health experts warn about electronic cigarettes [press release]. 2009 July 22, 2009 [cited 2009 August 12, 2009]; Available from: http://www.fda.gov/NewsEvents/Newsroom/PressAnnouncements/ucm173222.htm.

7. Canada, H., Notice: To all persons interested in importing, advertising or selling electronic smoking products in Canada. 2009.

8. Australian Government Department of Health and Ageing, N.D.a.P.S.C., *Record of Reasons, 54th Meeting*, 14-15 October 2008. 2008.

Chapter 16

Cigars And Pipes

Facts About Cigars

Cigars contain the same toxic and carcinogenic compounds found in cigarettes and are not a safe alternative to cigarettes. The three major types of cigars sold in the United States are large cigars, cigarillos, and little cigars. In 2007, cigar sales in the United States rose 9.2% and generated more than $3.4 billion in retail sales.

Health Effects

Regular cigar smoking is associated with an increased risk for cancers of the lung, oral cavity, larynx, and esophagus. Heavy cigar smokers and those who inhale deeply may be at increased risk for developing coronary heart disease and chronic obstructive pulmonary disease.

Current Estimates

- In 2007, an estimated 5.4%, or 13.3 million Americans, 12 years of age or older, were current cigar users.

- An estimated 7.3% of African American, 5.5% of white, 4.5% of Hispanic, 9.0% of American Indian/Alaska Native, and 1.4% of Asian American adults 18 years of age or older, are current cigar smokers.

About This Chapter: This chapter begins with text from "Cigars," Centers for Disease Control and Prevention, May 29, 2009. "Cigar Use among Young Adults Aged 18 to 25," is from *The NSDUH Report*, National Survey on Drug Use and Health, Substance Abuse and Mental Health Services Administration, January 15, 2009.

- An estimated 14.0% of students in grades 9–12 in the United States are current cigar smokers. Cigar smoking is more common among males (19.4%) than females (7.6%) in these grades.

- An estimated 4% of middle school students in the United States are current cigar smokers. Estimates are higher for middle school boys (5.3%) than girls (2.7%).

> ✤ **It's A Fact!!**
>
> - Nearly two thirds (65.9%) of young adults who used cigars in the past month also used cigarettes, 15.3% also used smokeless tobacco, and 5.8% also used pipe tobacco.
>
> Source: Substance Abuse and Mental Health Services Administration, January 15, 2009.

Other Information

- The two leading brands preferred by cigar smokers aged 12 years or older are Black & Mild® (22.8%) and Swisher Sweets® (14.4%).

- Marketing efforts have promoted cigars as symbols of a luxuriant and successful lifestyle. Endorsements by celebrities, development of cigar-friendly magazines (for example, *Cigar Aficionado*), features of highly visible women smoking cigars, and product placement in movies have contributed to the increased visibility of cigar smoking in society.

- Since 2001, cigar packaging and advertisements must display one of five health warning labels on a rotating basis.

Cigar Use Among Young Adults

This text examines past month cigar use among young adults aged 18 to 25, the age group with the highest rates of past month cigar use. The first section presents information on trends in cigar smoking from 2002 to 2007. The remaining sections use 2007 data to examine cigar use by demographic and geographic characteristics, and the prevalence of use of other types of tobacco among cigar users.

Trends In Past Month Cigar Use

More young adults used cigars in the past month in 2007 (11.8%) than in 2002 (11.0%), although the prevalence rate peaked in 2004 at 12.7%. Overall trends in past month cigar use were primarily driven by trends among males, who were generally three times as likely as females to have smoked cigars. In 2002, 16.8% of males used cigars compared to 19.7% in 2004 and 18.4% in 2007. Among females, rates remained relatively stable between 2002 and 2007, ranging from 5.1 to 5.8%.

Cigar Use By Demographic And Geographic Characteristics

In 2007, rates of past month cigar use varied by race/ethnicity and age group. The highest rate was found among young adults reporting two or more races (16.9%), followed by whites (13.4%), blacks or African Americans (11.2%), Hispanics or Latinos (8.3%), and Asians (4.4%). Rates of past month cigar use generally declined with age among young adults; for example, the rate was 14.5% for those aged 18 or 19 compared with 8.5% for those aged 24 or 25.

Rates also varied by geographic characteristics. Young adults living in non-metropolitan counties were more likely than those living in large or small metropolitan counties to have used cigars in the past month (13.5% vs. 11.4 and 11.8%). The rate of past month cigar use was higher among young adults living in the Midwest and the South (13.8 and 12.0%) than their counterparts living in the West and the Northeast (10.9 and 10.4%).

♣ It's A Fact!!

Although women don't smoke cigars and pipes as much as men, recent data show the number of women smoking cigars is increasing. Many people think that cigars and pipes are safer than cigarettes, but this is not true. Even if you don't inhale, you're still at higher risk for oral and throat cancers. Cigar and pipe smokers also have higher rates of lung cancer and heart disease than nonsmokers.

Source: Excerpted from "Smoking and How to Quit: Cigars and Pipes," National Women's Health Information Center (www.womenshealth.gov), June 17, 2009.

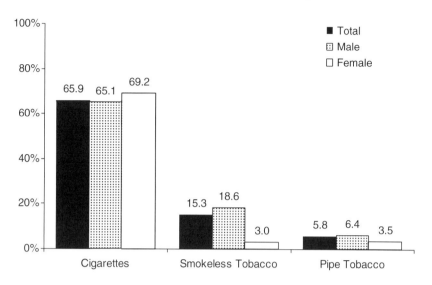

Figure 16.1. *Percentages of past month use of other tobacco products among past month cigar smokers aged 18 to 25, by gender—2007 (Source: SAMHSA, 2007 NSDUH).*

Use Of Other Tobacco Products Among Cigar Smokers

Nearly two thirds (65.9%) of past month cigar smokers also used cigarettes, 15.3% also used smokeless tobacco, and 5.8% also used pipe tobacco. Female and male past month cigarette use; however, males were more likely than females to have also used smokeless tobacco (18.6 vs. 3.0%) and pipe tobacco (6.4 vs. 3.5%).

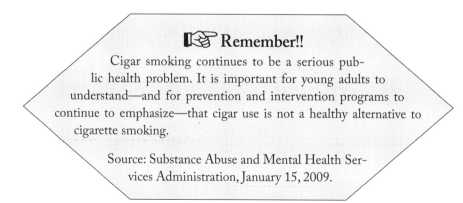

☞ Remember!!

Cigar smoking continues to be a serious public health problem. It is important for young adults to understand—and for prevention and intervention programs to continue to emphasize—that cigar use is not a healthy alternative to cigarette smoking.

Source: Substance Abuse and Mental Health Services Administration, January 15, 2009.

Chapter 17

Little Cigars And Cigarillos

What's the difference between cigarettes, little cigars, cigarillos, and cigars?

Cigarettes are wrapped in a paper tube. Anything with a tobacco wrapper is classified as a cigar. In the cigar group, the smallest are called "little cigars" (like Winchester or Cheyenne), the medium-sized ones are called "cigarillos" (like Black & Mild or Swisher Sweets), and the largest ones are usually just called "cigars."

The ingredients in these products may be a little different, but they're all filled with deadly, addictive tobacco.

Do these products have tobacco and nicotine?

Yes. They all have tobacco in them. Yes. They all have nicotine.

How bad are these products? Do they cause cancer?

Cigarillos and little cigars can be deadly. Just like cigarettes, smoking cigarillos and little cigars causes lung, mouth, and throat cancer and many other diseases.

About This Chapter: From "Answers about Black and Milds, Swisher Sweets, and Other Little Cigars and Cigarillos," by smokefree.gov (a website created by the Tobacco control Research Branch of the National Cancer Institute) and developed in collaboration with the American Legacy Foundation, 2008. The complete text of this article, including references, is available online at http://www.smokefree.gov/tob-cigarillo.aspx.

Are they addictive?

Yes. Nicotine is an addictive substance. Since little cigars and cigarillos all have nicotine, they all can be addictive.

Are cigarillos or little cigars safer than cigarettes?

No, cigarillos and little cigars can be as harmful as cigarettes. They can cause cancer and other diseases.

Aren't cigarillos more natural?

No. The basic ingredients are the same as in cigarettes. Sometimes cigarillos have flavorings added and have appealing scents, but they are still toxic.

Do people inhale cigarillos or little cigars? If they don't inhale, are they still dangerous?

Most cigar smokers don't inhale when they smoke, but some people inhale cigarillos and little cigars when they smoke them. Either way, they are harmful to your health and can cause cancer.

I've smoked a couple of cigarillos. Have I done a lot of damage?

Every puff of a cigarillo does more damage to your health and increases your chances of getting cancer. The more you smoke the more damage you do. The best thing is not to start smoking. If you already smoke, see the last question below for help quitting.

Is there anything I can do to make a cigar, little cigar, or cigarillo safer?

No. Whenever you inhale the smoke from burned tobacco, you are breathing in thousands of chemicals, some of

✎ What's It Mean?

Little cigars, cigarillos, and cigars include the following:

- Black and Mild, also called Black n Milds, Black & Milds, Blackies, Blacks, Milds, Tips, or Whiteheads

- Swisher Sweets, also called Swishers, or Sweets

- Dutch Masters, also called Dutches

- Phillies, White Owl, Captain Black, Prime Time, Winchesters, and Cheyenne

which cause cancer. And tobacco naturally has nicotine which is addictive so it can be very hard to stop smoking.

What percent of people smoke big cigars, little cigars, or cigarillos? Who smokes these?

About one in 20, or 5% of Americans smoke big cigars, little cigars, or cigarillos. A higher percentage of adults who haven't finished high school smoke cigars than those who have finished high school or college.

Why do some people take the paper out of Black and Milds (sometimes called freaking, champing, regulating, or hyping)? Does taking the paper out make them safer?

Some people take the liner paper out of the tube of cigarillos because they think it makes them less harsh or that it reduces the harm. But really, the tobacco inside is what causes cancer and other diseases.

Who makes these little cigars/cigarillos?

Most are made by a few large tobacco companies: Altadis, Altria (Philip Morris), Lane (R. J. Reynolds), Swedish Match, and Swisher.

Why do tobacco companies make so many different flavors of cigars and cigarillos?

Flavors may make these products more attractive to youth and adults who don't normally smoke.

Why are cigars sold on the counter but cigarettes are kept behind the counter? Why can you buy a single cigarillo but not a single cigarette?

There are different laws for cigarettes and cigarillos about how they can be packaged and sold.

Are menthol cigarillos safer than non-menthol cigarillos?

No. Adding menthol to tobacco does not make it safer. Even though people may think that they are less harsh, they still cause cancer.

Are tobacco companies directing their ads at African-Americans?

Research says yes. Studies show that there are more than twice as many tobacco ads per person in African-American neighborhoods than white ones. This is particularly alarming, since there are more tobacco-related deaths among African-Americans than among whites.

I want to quit smoking little cigars or cigarillos. Where can I go to get help?

Here are some websites where you can learn how to quit:

- http://www.smokefree.gov
- http://www.becomeanex.org

Or you can get free help quitting from a live person by calling: 800-QUIT-NOW (784-8669).

✔ Quick Tip

You can learn more about tobacco use prevention at these websites:

http://www.thetruth.com

http://www.tobaccofreekids.org

Chapter 18

Bidis And Kreteks

Contrary to popular belief, clove cigarettes, also called kreteks, contain tobacco—they are made up of 60–70 percent tobacco and 30–40 percent shredded cloves (a spice). Considering their tobacco content, clove cigarettes are probably as harmful and dangerous as regular cigarettes. As a matter of fact, kreteks may hold even more risk than ordinary smokes. According to the U.S. Centers for Disease Control and Prevention (CDC), clove cigarettes produce at least twice as much nicotine, tar, and carbon monoxide as regular American cigarettes brands.

Plus, there may be an additional risk due to their clove content. The major active ingredient in cloves is eugenol, which is a topical anesthetic used in dentistry. The short- and long-term health effects of eugenol are not well known, and little inhalation toxicology research has been done on this substance. However, when smoked, eugenol numbs the throat and impairs the gag reflex. This anesthetizing effect could cause some problems; for example, liquids and/or food could more easily go down the wrong pipe. Smokers may not feel the harshness of the smoke as strongly, so they are more likely to inhale the smoke more deeply and hold it in the lungs for a longer period of time before exhaling. As a result, it's

About This Chapter: This chapter begins with information reprinted with permission from Go Ask Alice!, Columbia University's Health Q&A Internet Resource, at www.goaskalice .columbia.edu. Copyright © 2009 by The Trustees of Columbia University. Additional information about Go Ask Alice materials is included at the end of this chapter. Text under the headings "Health Effects of Bidis and Kreteks" and "Current U.S. Estimates of Bidis and Kreteks Use" is excerpted from "Bidis and Kreteks" Centers for Disease Control and Prevention, May 29, 2009.

possible, or even likely, that eugenol has the potential to facilitate lung infections, respiratory illnesses, or allergic reactions in certain users, especially in smokers with existing breathing problems and/or other sensitivities.

Although clove cigarette smokers share some adverse health symptoms, such as nausea, vomiting, allergic reactions, bronchitis, pneumonia, and coughing up blood, the cause-and-effect relationship between smoking clove cigarettes and these symptoms has not yet been definitively established. Regardless, it seems reasonable to assume that clove cigarettes are as harmful and dangerous or even more so than standard cigarettes.

Clove cigarettes are one of several kinds of alternative smokes. Others include bidis (tiny, inexpensive, flavored dark tobacco containing cigarettes hand rolled with a dried tendu leaf), herbal or vegetable-based cigarettes with no tobacco and nicotine, and additive-free, natural tobacco cigarettes. Often, alternative cigarette smokers are part of the under 30 crowd. People smoke the "alternatives" because they think that they are cool and/or safer, healthier, and more natural to smoke than standard smokes. Cool or not, smoking alternative cigarettes can be as harmful and even dangerous to one's health as regular ones.

Health Effects Of Bidis And Kreteks

Research studies on the health effects of bidis have not been conducted in the United States. Research studies from India indicate that bidi smoking is associated with an increased risk for oral cancer as well as an increased risk for cancer of the lung, stomach, and esophagus.

Research studies in India show that bidi smoking is associated with a more than three-fold increased risk for coronary heart disease and acute myocardial infarction (heart attack) and a nearly four-fold increased risk for chronic bronchitis.

Kretek smoking is associated with an increased risk for acute lung injury, especially among susceptible individuals with asthma or respiratory infections.

Research studies on the long-term health effects of kreteks have not been conducted in the United States. Research in Indonesia shows that regular kretek smokers have 13–20 times the risk for abnormal lung function compared with nonsmokers.

✎ What's It Mean?

"Natural" cigarettes include clove cigarettes, also called kreteks (kree-teks), and flavored cigarettes, called "bidis" or "beedies." Both cigarette types are imported mainly from Southeast Asian countries. In addition to tobacco, they contain various flavorings. Kreteks contain ground cloves and clove oil. Bidis contain candy-like flavors, such as chocolate, cherry, and mango.

Some young people think that kreteks and bidis are safer than regular cigarettes because of the "natural" flavorings. Also, the packs often do not have warning labels. In fact, both kreteks and bidis deliver more nicotine, tar, and carbon monoxide than regular cigarettes. Like smoking regular cigarettes, smoking kreteks and bidis can cause cancer and other diseases.

Another type of "natural" cigarette is the herbal cigarette. This is made from a blend of herbs, such as passion flower, jasmine, and ginseng. Although herbal cigarettes contain no tobacco or nicotine, the smoke contains tar, carbon monoxide, and other toxins. As a result, herbal cigarettes can be dangerous to your health.

Source: Excerpted from "Smoking and How to Quit: "Natural" Cigarettes," National Women's Health Information Center (www.womenshealth.gov), June 17, 2009.

Current U.S. Estimates Of Bidis And Kreteks Use

- There are no national estimates for bidi or kretek smoking among adults in the United States.

- An estimated three percent of high school students are current bidi smokers. Bidi smoking is more than twice as common among male (four percent) compared with female (two percent) high school students.

- An estimated two percent of middle school students are current bidi smokers. Bidi smoking is more common among male (three percent) compared with female (two percent) middle school students.

- An estimated three percent of high school students are current kretek smokers. Kretek smoking is more common among male (three percent) than female (two percent) high school students.

• An estimated two percent of middle school students are current kretek smokers. Kretek use is more common among male (two percent) compared with female (one percent) middle school students.

Regarding Information From Go Ask Alice

Information within this chapter marked © 2009 by the Trustees of Columbia University is protected by copyright owned in whole or in principal part by The Trustees of Columbia University in the City of New York ("Columbia"). You may copy the document for reference and research purposes only. Columbia makes no representations or warranties, express or implied, with respect to the document, or any part thereof, including any warranties of title, noninfringement of copyright or patent rights of others, merchantability, or fitness or suitability for any purpose.

Distribution and/or alteration by not-for-profit research or educational institutions for their local use is permitted as long as this notice is kept intact and attached to the document. Any other distribution of copies of the document or any altered version thereof is expressly prohibited without prior written consent of Columbia.

Chapter 19

Hookah Pipes

What Hookahs Are And How They Work

They come in a variety of designs, sizes, materials, and colors, but typical hookahs have the following components:

- A bowl where the tobacco is placed and heated, usually with burning embers or charcoal,

- A vase or smoke chamber which is partially filled with water,

- A pipe or stem connecting the bowl to the vase by a tube that carries the smoke down into the water, and

- A hose with a mouthpiece through which the smoke is drawn from the vase.

About This Chapter: Excerpted from "Reducing Hookah Use: A Public Health Challenge for the 21st Century," © 2007 The BACCHUS Network. Reprinted with permission. The complete report, including references, is available at http://www.tobaccofreeu.org/pdf/HookahWhitePaper.pdf. The BACCHUS Network™, a 501 C3 non-profit organization, actively promotes student, campus and community-wide leadership on healthy and safe lifestyle decisions through peer-to-peer education. The BACCHUS philosophy is that students can play a uniquely effective role—unmatched by professional educators—in encouraging their peers to consider, talk honestly about and develop responsible habits and attitudes toward health and safety issues. BACCHUS and its nearly 1,000 campus-based affiliates focus on topics ranging from alcohol abuse, tobacco use, unhealthy sexual practices, illegal drug issues, mental health concerns, fitness and nutrition. For additional information, visit www.bacchusnetwork.org or www.tobaccofreeU.org.

As the smoker inhales, the tobacco smoke is sucked down from the bowl and then bubbles up through the water into the air of the smoke chamber and then through the hose to the smoker. The water in the vase cools the smoke and filters out some of its tar and particulates. At the end of a smoking session, the dirty water is thrown away and the hookah vase refilled for the next user or users. Most smoking sessions last from 45 to 60 minutes but they can continue for several hours.

While hookah is the most common word used among English speakers, other terms used include narghile or nargile, goza, ghalyun, and hubble bubble. Hookahs are made with single hoses or three or more of them connected to the base for multiple users. Hookahs are made with a variety of materials and come in a variety of colors. Many of them have been made into works of art by skilled craftsmen in India, Iran, Turkey, and the Middle East.

Hookah History And Culture

Hookah smoking may have originated in India and then spread to Persia, Afghanistan, the Middle East, Turkey, and Africa. Hookahs were first used to smoke opium or hashish, but during the late 16th and early 17th centuries, they became much more popular with the introduction of tobacco from America and the opening of multiple public coffee houses. Hookahs became a central feature of coffee house culture with users spending hours with friends in cafes smoking, drinking mint tea or coffee, and/or playing chess, dominoes, or backgammon.

✎ What's It Mean?

Hookahs—sometimes called water pipes—are used to smoke specially made tobacco. Hookah tobacco is available in a variety of flavors, such as apple, mint, cherry, chocolate, coconut, licorice, cappuccino, and watermelon. Hookah smoking is typically practiced in groups, with the same mouthpiece passed from person to person. Hookahs are known by a number of different names, including narghile, argileh, shisha, hubble-bubble, and goza.

Source: Excerpted from "Hookahs," Centers for Disease Control and Prevention, September 2009.

Over the years, hookahs became embedded in the traditional cultures of Turkey, the Middle East, Iran, Afghanistan, India and parts of Africa. Hookah use was a ceremonial activity governed by strict rules for each stage in the process of preparing, lighting, and smoking. Refusal to share your hookah with a guest was considered a grave insult. Most Middle Eastern hookah smokers were adult males and older females, but hookahs also became popular among upper-class Turkish women who offered them to guests with afternoon tea and at intellectual gatherings.

During the past century hookah use declined as cigarettes became more widely available. Most hookah smokers were elderly and retired men who congregated in bazaar cafes in poor neighborhoods. Since the 1990s, however, hookah use has rapidly expanded, spreading from the Middle East to other parts of the world including the U.S.

♣ It's A Fact!!
Correcting Myths About Hookah Smoking

- It is not safer than smoking cigarettes. Hookah smokers are exposed to cancer-causing chemicals and hazardous gases such as carbon monoxide. Hookah is linked to lung, oral and bladder cancer, as well as clogged arteries and heart disease.

- Hookah is addictive. People ingest higher nicotine levels than with cigarettes, which could increase the risk of addiction since nicotine is the drug that causes addiction.

- The water pipe does not filter out the "bad stuff". The water-filtration and extended hose does not filter out the nicotine, tar, cancer-causing chemicals, and dangerous heavy metals.

- Smokers who share a water pipe are at risk for infectious diseases, such as tuberculosis, and viruses such as hepatitis and herpes. Shared mouthpieces may enhance the opportunity for such diseases to spread.

Source: Excerpted from "How to Talk to Teens about Dangerous Hookah (Water Pipe) Smoking," and reprinted with permission from the Rhode Island Department of Health Office for Family, Youth and School Success (http://www.health.ri.gov/family/ofyss). © 2007 Rhode Island Department of Health.

Prevalence

Most of the data on hookah use prevalence are from Middle Eastern studies. Results from a representative sample of these studies indicate that:

- 19% of 635 young Egyptian teenagers had used hookahs.

- 41% of 388 Israeli schoolchildren aged 12 to 18 years smoked hookahs, and 22% of these users smoked every weekend.

- Of 587 Syrian university students, 63% of the men and 30% of the women had ever used hookahs: currently, 26% of the men and 5% of the women still used them.

- Among 1,964 Lebanese university students in a 2001 survey, 31% of the men and 23% of the women used hookahs weekly.

- 57% of men and 69% of women in a national survey of 4,000 Kuwaiti government workers had used hookahs at least once.

- The percentage of American University of Beirut students who had ever used a hookah rose from 30% in 1998 to 43% in 2002.

Prevalence data on hookah use in the U.S. are limited to a survey of 1,671 teens (mostly Arab-American) aged 14 to 18 years and living in Michigan. Among study participants, 27% had used hookahs and the percentage of users increased from 23% at age 14 to 40% at age 18. Hookah users were twice as likely as non-users to be smoking cigarettes as well and that the odds of experimenting with cigarettes were eight times as high for anyone who had ever used a hookah as for non-users. In this country, the use of hookahs has become increasingly widespread with the growing numbers of Arab immigrants and Arab-Americans and increasingly popular among youth and young adults in the general population.

Two surveys of 300 students each conducted in 2005 and 2006 by Breathe California, Sacramento, found that during the first year, 45% of the students had used hookahs during the past two months. In 2006, 40% of the students were at events where hookahs were used and of these, 58% used hookahs during the past six months.

In the spring of 2007, campus professionals and national young adult tobacco control experts were interviewed about their perception of hookah use and youth and young adults. Most interview participants reported growing numbers of middle school, high school, and college students smoking with hookahs in their communities and across the country. Also reported were a proliferation of hookah bars and growing numbers of students smoking hookahs with friends inside or outside their residence halls, in their apartments or houses. Hookahs have became a common topic of conversation among students. Expanding hookah use has also been reported by the media.

Why Hookahs Have Become So Popular

Major reasons for the growing popularity of hookah use worldwide since the 1990s include the introduction of a flavored tobacco mix, the mushrooming of hookah establishments, aggressive marketing, and media hype about this new trend.

❖ It's A Fact!!

Middle Eastern men have smoked hookah pipes for hundreds of years. Now, this form of smoking is becoming popular in the United States, especially among young people. A hookah is a water pipe that holds tobacco. The tobacco is often mixed with honey, molasses, or dried fruit to give flavoring to the smoke. When a person inhales on a hose attached to the hookah, the smoke is filtered through water in the base. Passing the smoke through the water partially filters tar and small particles from the smoke.

Because the pipe filters the tobacco smoke, hookahs are advertised as safer than cigarettes. In fact, hookah smoke contains levels of nicotine, carbon monoxide, and tar that are as high or higher than those found in the smoke from many filtered cigarettes. Several types of cancer, as well as gum disease, have been linked to hookah smoking.

Source: Excerpted from "Smoking and How to Quit: Hookah Pipes," National Women's Health Information Center (www.womenshealth.gov), June 17, 2009.

Introduction Of Flavored Tobacco

In the early 1990s, Egyptian tobacco companies introduced "Maassel," a specially prepared mixture containing sweetened fruit flavors and mild aromatic smoke which has helped to attract new hookah users worldwide. Maassel, known as "shisha" in the U.S., consists of about 30% of crude cut tobacco fermented with about 70% of honey, molasses, and the pulp of different fruits. It provides a pleasant aroma when heated slowly with burning charcoal and comes in a variety of flavors including apple, strawberry, rose, mango, cappuccino, banana, peach, lemon, orange, mint, and licorice. Currently, most hookah smokers around the world use Maassel rather than the traditional tobacco mix because it is more flavorful and makes the process of waterpipe preparation simpler because users do not need to moisten, shape, and dry the tobacco before use, as with other kinds of tobacco like Ajami.

Hookah Bars, Cafes, And Restaurants

Hookah bars, cafes, and restaurants have become popular social gathering places for young smokers and their friends and their numbers have increased dramatically in recent years. In the U.S., the estimated number of these establishments now ranges from 300 to 1,000. Directories listing hookah bars and cafes in large cities and the States are posted on the internet and these places are touted in the media. BACCHUS survey participants reported large increases in the numbers of hookah establishments in their communities during the past several years, for example, from two to 25 in Denver, from zero to four in Fort Collins, Colorado, and from zero to seven in Sacramento.

Hookah bars, cafes, and restaurants lure customers through advertising in college/university and local newspapers, radio stations popular among young people, and by emphasizing exotic aspects of Middle Eastern culture in their décor, furnishings, music, and displays of a variety of colorful, finely crafted hookahs. These places especially appeal to some college students under the age of 21 because they do not serve alcoholic beverages.

Aggressive Marketing

Multiple enterprises have sprung up in the U.S. and Middle East to take advantage of a booming business fueled by aggressive marketing of hookahs, hookah accessories, and Maassel. For example, in Bahrain, revenues from hookah tobacco exports to other Middle-Eastern countries increased by 9% to about $25 million from 1995 to 1996. Most of the "shisha" imported to the U.S. comes from companies in the United Arab Emirates, Jordan, Egypt, and Saudi Arabia. The owner of the Florida-based website recently reported that the demand for hookahs was at an all-time high and that sales were highest in California, Arizona, New York, Texas, and Virginia. A Detroit wholesaler also made more than $1 million in sales the previous year to tobacco shops, hookah cafes and stores across the country and predicted that sales would triple in the coming year.

Many businesses have developed websites to advertise their hookah products. To attract customers, these businesses offer a variety of hookahs for sale, for example, Egyptian Hookahs, Sheik Hookahs, Rotating Hookahs, and Modern Hookahs or give these products exotic names like "Scheherazade," "Syrian Queen," and "Queen Nefertiti." Other websites promote hookah use as chic and elegant or as part of a unique lifestyle and hookahs as objects of religious veneration.

Media Hype

The media (radio, satellite TV, and the press) has also helped to boost the global expansion of hookah use by glamorizing this practice. U.S. newspaper reporters depict hookah use as new, trendy, and safe for college students and other young people, although some of them do warn about its potential health effects. Most of the BACCHUS survey participants reported reading articles in campus and local newspapers promoting hookah use. For example, one article in the *Colorado State University's Rocky Mountain Collegian* reports that when a student first walked into a hookah bar she was "instantly hooked." Also, an editorial in this paper, praised the Fort Collins city council for granting local hookah bars exemptions from the local ordinance prohibiting smoking in public places.

Health Risks Of Hookah Use

Assessing the specific dangers of hookah use is challenging because some users also smoke cigarettes; the extent to which it is harmful likely depends on the duration and frequency of use, and there is wide variation in the content of the different brands of hookah tobacco.

✤ It's A Fact!!
Hookah Smoke And Cancer

- The charcoal used to heat tobacco in the hookah increases the health risks by producing high levels of carbon monoxide, metals, and cancer-causing chemicals.

- Even after it has passed through water, the smoke produced by a hookah contains high levels of toxic compounds, including carbon monoxide, heavy metals, and cancer-causing chemicals.

- Hookah tobacco and smoke contain numerous toxic substances known to cause lung, bladder, and oral cancers.

- Irritation from exposure to tobacco juices increases the risk of developing oral cancers. The irritation by tobacco juice products is likely to be greater among hookah smokers than among pipe or cigar smokers because hookah smoking is typically practiced (with or without inhalation) more often and for longer periods of time.

Other Health Effects Of Hookah Smoke

- Hookah tobacco and smoke contain numerous toxic substances known to cause clogged arteries and heart disease.

- Sharing a hookah may increase the risk of transmitting tuberculosis, viruses such as herpes or hepatitis, and other illnesses.

- Babies born to women who smoked one or more water pipes a day during pregnancy have lower birth weights (were at least 3½ ounces less) than babies born to nonsmokers and are at an increased risk for respiratory diseases.

- Secondhand smoke from hookahs poses a serious risk for nonsmokers, particularly because it contains smoke from the tobacco and smoke from the heat source (for example, charcoal) used in the hookah.

Source: Excerpted from "Hookahs," Centers for Disease Control and Prevention, September 2009.

Constituents Of Hookah Smoke

Despite these challenges, studies provide ample evidence that hookah smoking is not a safe alternative to cigarette smoking. Hookah smoke has been found to contain high concentrations of carbon monoxide (CO), nicotine, "tar", and heavy metals. Also, commonly used heat sources like charcoal or wood cinders may increase health risks because they produce such toxicants as CO, metals, and carcinogens. These risks may be increased by using quick-burning charcoal which likely emits more CO than the charcoal traditionally used in the Middle East.

Health Effects

Health problems identified by researchers in the Middle East, China, and India include lung, oral and bladder cancer, and cancer of the esophagus and stomach; heart disease; and respiratory problems. Other health risks include nicotine dependence and infections like tuberculosis, herpes, and hepatitis which can be transmitted through the sharing of the same mouthpiece—a common custom in many cultures. BACCHUS survey participants expressed concern that hookah use by teens and young adults would serve as a gateway to cigarette smoking in later years. Two participants also reported an outbreak of mononucleosis in Denver among young hookah bar customers who had shared mouthpieces. They noted that hookah bars are not required to sterilize or replace these mouthpieces after use.

Health Risks For Children

Women using hookahs during pregnancy may expose their unborn children to low birth weight, low Apgar scores and respiratory distress. Children exposed to secondhand smoke (SHS) from hookahs at home may suffer from respiratory ailments and also from similar problems as children whose families smoke cigarettes, for example, ear and upper respiratory infection, asthma, and sudden infant death syndrome.

Chapter 20

Smokeless Tobacco

Smokeless Tobacco and Cancer: Questions and Answers

Snuff is a finely ground or shredded tobacco that is either sniffed through the nose or placed between the cheek and gum. Chewing tobacco is used by putting a wad of tobacco inside the cheek. Chewing tobacco and snuff contain 28 cancer-causing agents. Smokeless tobacco users have an increased risk of developing cancer of the oral cavity. Several national organizations offer information about the health risks of smokeless tobacco and how to quit.

What is smokeless tobacco?

There are two types of smokeless tobacco—snuff and chewing tobacco. Snuff, a finely ground or shredded tobacco, is packaged as dry, moist, or in sachets (tea bag–like pouches). Typically, the user places a pinch or dip between the cheek and gum. Chewing tobacco is available in loose leaf, plug (plug-firm and plug-moist), or twist forms, with the user putting a wad of tobacco inside the cheek. Smokeless tobacco is sometimes called "spit" or "spitting" tobacco because people spit out the tobacco juices and saliva that build up in the mouth.

About This Chapter: This chapter includes text from "Smokeless Tobacco and Cancer: Questions and Answers," National Cancer Institute, May 30, 2003; and "Smokeless Tobacco Use, Initiation, and Relationship to Cigarette Smoking: 2002 to 2007," *The NSDUH Report*, National Survey on Drug Use and Human Health, Substance Abuse and Mental Health Services Administration, March 5, 2009.

What harmful chemicals are found in smokeless tobacco?

Chewing tobacco and snuff contain 28 carcinogens (cancer-causing agents). The most harmful carcinogens in smokeless tobacco are the tobacco-specific nitrosamines (TSNAs). They are formed during the growing, curing, fermenting, and aging of tobacco. TSNAs have been detected in some smokeless tobacco products at levels many times higher than levels of other types of nitrosamines that are allowed in foods, such as bacon and beer.

Other cancer-causing substances in smokeless tobacco include N-nitrosamino acids, volatile N-nitrosamines, benzo(a)pyrene, volatile aldehydes, formaldehyde, acetaldehyde, crotonaldehyde, hydrazine, arsenic, nickel, cadmium, benzopyrene, and polonium-210.

What cancers are caused by or associated with smokeless tobacco use?

Smokeless tobacco users increase their risk for cancer of the oral cavity. Oral cancer can include cancer of the lip, tongue, cheeks, gums, and the floor and roof of the mouth.

People who use oral snuff for a long time have a much greater risk for cancer of the cheek and gum than people who do not use smokeless tobacco.

♣ **It's A Fact!!**

All tobacco, including smokeless tobacco, contains nicotine, which is addictive. The amount of nicotine absorbed from smokeless tobacco is three to four times the amount delivered by a cigarette. Nicotine is absorbed more slowly from smokeless tobacco than from cigarettes, but more nicotine per dose is absorbed from smokeless tobacco than from cigarettes. Also, the nicotine stays in the bloodstream for a longer time.

Source: Excerpted from "Smokeless Tobacco and Cancer: Questions and Answers," National Cancer Institute, May 30, 2003.

The possible increased risk for other types of cancer from smokeless tobacco is being studied.

What are some of the other ways smokeless tobacco can harm users' health?

Some of the other effects of smokeless tobacco use include addiction to nicotine, oral leukoplakia (white mouth lesions that can become cancerous), gum disease, and gum recession (when the gum pulls away from the teeth). Possible increased risks for heart disease, diabetes, and reproductive problems are being studied.

Is smokeless tobacco a good substitute for cigarettes?

In 1986, the Surgeon General concluded that the use of smokeless tobacco "is not a safe substitute for smoking cigarettes. It can cause cancer and a number of noncancerous conditions and can lead to nicotine addiction and dependence." Since 1991, the National Cancer Institute (NCI), a part of the National Institutes of Health, has officially recommended that the public avoid and discontinue the use of all tobacco products, including smokeless tobacco. NCI also recognizes that nitrosamines, found in tobacco products, are not safe at any level. The accumulated scientific evidence does not support changing this position.

Who uses smokeless tobacco?

In the United States, the 2000 National Household Survey on Drug Abuse, which was conducted by the Substance Abuse and Mental Health Services Administration, reported the following statistics:

- An estimated 7.6 million Americans age 12 and older (3.4%) had used smokeless tobacco in the past month.

- Smokeless tobacco use was most common among young adults ages 18 to 25.

- Men were 10 times more likely than women to report using smokeless tobacco (6.5% of men age 12 and older compared with 0.5% of women).

People in many other countries and regions, including India, parts of Africa, and some Central Asian countries, have a long history of using smokeless tobacco products.

> **✔ Quick Tip**
> ## What about using smokeless tobacco to quit cigarettes?
>
> Because all tobacco use causes disease and addiction, National Cancer Institute recommends that tobacco use be avoided and discontinued. Several nontobacco methods have been shown to be effective for quitting cigarettes. These methods include pharmacotherapies such as nicotine replacement therapy and bupropion, individual and group counseling, and telephone quitlines.
>
> Source: Excerpted from "Smokeless Tobacco and Cancer: Questions and Answers," National Cancer Institute, May 30, 2003.

Smokeless Tobacco Use, Initiation, and Relationship to Cigarette Smoking

The National Survey on Drug Use and Health (NSDUH) asks persons aged 12 or older about their substance use, including their use of tobacco products. The questions on tobacco products focus on cigarettes, cigars, pipe tobacco, and smokeless tobacco (that is, chewing tobacco and snuff). Respondents who used these substances are asked when they first used them.

This text examines smokeless tobacco use and its relationship to cigarette smoking among persons aged 12 or older. The first section presents information on trends in the use of smokeless tobacco using NSDUH data from 2002 to 2007. Unless otherwise noted, all other findings are annual averages based on data from the combined 2002 to 2007 surveys.

Trends In Smokeless Tobacco Use And Initiation Of Use

Among persons aged 12 or older, past month smokeless tobacco use remained relatively stable in the range of 3.0 to 3.3% between 2002 and 2007. This finding was consistent across most gender and age groups. However, among males aged 12 to 17, past month smokeless tobacco use increased significantly—from 3.4% in 2002 to 4.4% in 2007. Among persons aged 12 or older, the rate of recent initiation of smokeless tobacco use (that is, first-time use of smokeless tobacco in the 12 months before the survey interview among all persons who had not previously used it) showed a modest, but statistically significant increase between 2002 and 2007 (from 0.5 to 0.6%) (Table 20.1). Initiation rates were higher in 2007 than in 2002 among males aged 12 to 17 and males aged 18 to 25. Among females, there were no statistically significant changes in initiation rates for any age group over the 6-year period.

Table 20.1. Percentages of persons aged 12 or older initiating smokeless tobacco use in the past year among those eligible for initiation, by age group and gender—2002 to 2007

Age Group/Gender	2002	2003	2004	2005	2006	2007
Total	0.5	0.5	0.5	0.6	0.7	0.6
Aged 12 to 17						
Male	3.0	3.4	2.9	3.5	3.9	4.0
Female	1.0	0.8	0.9	1.1	1.0	1.2
Aged 18 to 25						
Male	3.1	2.5	2.9	3.4	3.9	3.9
Female	0.6	0.6	0.8	0.8	0.7	0.9
Aged 26 or Older						
Male	0.1	0.1	0.1	0.1	0.2	0.1
Female	0.0	0.0	0.1	0.0	0.1	0.1

Source: SAMHSA, 2002 to 2007 NSDUHs.

Smokeless Tobacco Use, By Demographic And Geographic Characteristics

Combined 2002 to 2007 data indicate that an annual average of 3.2% of persons aged 12 or older (an estimated 7.8 million persons) used smokeless tobacco in the past month. Certain demographic subgroups were more likely to use smokeless tobacco than others. It was more likely to be used among persons aged 18 to 25 than among 12 to 17 year olds and those 26 or older (Table 20.2). Males were more likely than females to have used smokeless tobacco (6.2 vs. 0.4%). American Indians or Alaska Natives were more likely than persons in any other racial/ethnic category to have used smokeless tobacco.

Rates also varied by geographic characteristics. Past month smokeless tobacco use was highest among persons who lived in completely rural and less urbanized counties in non-metropolitan areas and lowest among persons who lived in large metropolitan areas. Persons who lived in the South and Midwest were more likely than person who lived in the West and Northeast to have used smokeless tobacco.

Table 20.2. Percentages of persons aged 12 or older using smokeless tobacco in the past month, by demographic and geographic characteristics—2002 to 2007

Demographic and Geographic Characteristic	Past Month	Demographic and Geographic Characteristic	Past Month
Age Group in Years		**County Type**	
12 to 17	2.2	Large Metropolitan	1.9
18 to 25	5.0	Small Metropolitan	3.7
26 or Older	3.0	250,000 to 1 Million Population	3.2
Gender		<250,000 Population	4.7
Male	6.2	Non-Metropolitan	6.6
Female	0.4	Urbanized	5.5
Race/Ethnicity		Less Urbanized	7.1
White	4.1	Completely Rural	8.4
Black or African American	1.4	**Region**	
American Indian or Alaska Native	7.1	Northeast	1.7
Native Hawaiian or Other Pacific Islander	2.9	Midwest	3.7
Asian	0.6	South	4.2
Hispanic or Latino	0.9	West	2.4
Two or More Races	2.9		

Source: SAMHSA, 2002 to 2007 NSDUHs.

Initiation Of Smokeless Tobacco Use, By Demographic Characteristics

Combined data from 2002 to 2007 indicate that an annual average of 1.1 million persons initiated use of smokeless tobacco in the past 12 months. This represents 0.6% of those at risk for initiation (that is, those who had not previously used smokeless tobacco). Initiation of smokeless tobacco in the past 12 months was more likely to occur among youths aged 12 to 17 than among young adults aged 18 to 25 (2.2 vs. 1.8%). Both of these age groups had higher rates of initiation than adults aged 26 or older (0.1%). Among those at risk for initiation of smokeless tobacco use, the rate of recent initiation was higher among males than females (1.0 vs. 0.2%).

Cigarette Use Among Smokeless Tobacco Users

Combined data from 2002 to 2007 indicate that 85.8% of past month smokeless tobacco users used cigarettes at some time in their lives, and 38.8% used cigarettes in the past month. The rate of current cigarette use was 66.9% among past month smokeless tobacco users aged 18 to 25, 52.8% among those aged 12 to 17, and 29.3% among those aged 26 or older.

☞ Remember!!

Smokeless tobacco contains 28 cancer-causing agents and has been linked to oral cancer and increased risk of death from cardiovascular diseases. Chewing tobacco leads to nicotine dependence, as does cigarette use. The information reported in this chapter indicates that although rates of use remained stable between 2002 and 2007, there were increases among certain subpopulations—in particular, among adolescent males. Most smokeless tobacco users smoked cigarettes at some time in their lives, and most people who used both cigarettes and smokeless tobacco had used cigarettes first. It is important for current and former cigarette users to understand that smokeless tobacco use is not a healthy alternative to cigarette smoking.

Source: Substance Abuse and Mental Health Services Administration, March 5, 2009.

Initiation And Cessation Patterns For Smokeless Tobacco And Cigarettes

Combined 2004 to 2007 data indicate that, among persons who had used both smokeless tobacco and cigarettes in their lifetime, 31.8% started using smokeless tobacco first, 65.5% started using cigarettes first, and 2.7% initiated use of smokeless tobacco and cigarettes at about the same time (that is, within the same month). Nearly half (47.0%) of past month smokeless tobacco users were former cigarette users (that is, used cigarettes at some time in the past, but not in the past month). Some initiates of smokeless tobacco use may be cigarette smokers who are substituting smokeless tobacco as a way to quit smoking. Among daily smokers who initiated smokeless tobacco use, 88.1% were still smoking daily six months later.

Chapter 21

Secondhand Smoke

While secondhand smoke has been referred to as environmental tobacco smoke (ETS) in the past, the term "secondhand" smoke better captures the involuntary nature of the exposure. The 2006 Surgeon General's report uses the term "involuntary" in the title because most nonsmokers do not want to breathe tobacco smoke. The term "involuntary" was also used in the title of the 1986 Surgeon General's report on secondhand smoke.

Cigarette smoke contains more than 4,000 chemical compounds, many of the same chemicals that are present in the smoke inhaled by smokers. Because sidestream smoke is generated at lower temperatures and under different conditions than mainstream smoke, however, it contains higher concentrations of many of the toxins found in cigarette smoke.

The National Toxicology Program estimates that at least 250 chemicals in secondhand smoke are known to be toxic or carcinogenic, and the Surgeon General has concluded that there is no risk-free level of exposure to secondhand smoke: even small amounts of secondhand smoke exposure can be harmful to people's health. Many millions of Americans continue to be exposed to secondhand smoke. A smoke-free environment is the only way to

About This Chapter: From *The Health Consequences of Involuntary Exposure to Tobacco Smoke: A Report of the Surgeon General*, U.S. Department of Health and Human Services, January 4, 2007.

fully protect nonsmokers from the dangers of secondhand smoke. Separating smokers from nonsmokers, cleaning the air, and ventilating buildings cannot eliminate exposure of nonsmokers to secondhand smoke.

Six Major Conclusions Of The Surgeon General Report

Smoking is the single greatest avoidable cause of disease and death. In the report, *The Health Consequences of Involuntary Exposure to Tobacco Smoke: A Report of the Surgeon General,* the Surgeon General has concluded that any millions of Americans, both children and adults, are still exposed to second-hand smoke in their homes and workplaces despite substantial progress in tobacco control.

- Levels of a chemical called cotinine, a biomarker of secondhand smoke exposure, fell by 70% from 1988–91 to 2001–02. In national surveys, however, 43% of U.S. nonsmokers still have detectable levels of cotinine.

- Almost 60% of U.S. children aged 3–11 years—or almost 22 million children—are exposed to secondhand smoke.

- Approximately 30% of indoor workers in the United States are not covered by smoke-free workplace policies.

✎ What's It Mean?

Secondhand Smoke: Secondhand smoke (also called environmental tobacco smoke) is the combination of sidestream smoke (the smoke given off by the burning end of a tobacco product) and mainstream smoke (the smoke exhaled by the smoker). Exposure to secondhand smoke is also called involuntary smoking or passive smoking. People are exposed to secondhand smoke in homes, cars, the workplace, and public places such as bars, restaurants, and other recreation settings. In the United States, the source of most secondhand smoke is from cigarettes, followed by pipes, cigars, and other tobacco products.

Source: Excerpted from "Secondhand Smoke: Questions and Answers," National Cancer Institute, August 1, 2007.

Secondhand smoke exposure causes disease and premature death in children and adults who do not smoke.

- Secondhand smoke contains hundreds of chemicals known to be toxic or carcinogenic (cancer-causing), including formaldehyde, benzene, vinyl chloride, arsenic, ammonia, and hydrogen cyanide.

- Secondhand smoke has been designated as a known human carcinogen (cancer-causing agent) by the U.S. Environmental Protection Agency, National Toxicology Program and the International Agency for Research on Cancer (IARC). The National Institute for Occupational Safety and Health has concluded that secondhand smoke is an occupational carcinogen.

Children exposed to secondhand smoke are at an increased risk for sudden infant death syndrome (SIDS), acute respiratory infections, ear problems, and more severe asthma. Smoking by parents causes respiratory symptoms and slows lung growth in their children.

- Children who are exposed to secondhand smoke are inhaling many of the same cancer-causing substances and poisons as smokers. Because their bodies are developing, infants and young children are especially vulnerable to the poisons in secondhand smoke.

- Both babies whose mothers smoke while pregnant and babies who are exposed to secondhand smoke after birth are more likely to die from sudden infant death syndrome (SIDS) than babies who are not exposed to cigarette smoke.

- Babies whose mothers smoke while pregnant or who are exposed to secondhand smoke after birth have weaker lungs than unexposed babies, which increases the risk for many health problems.

- Among infants and children, secondhand smoke cause bronchitis and pneumonia, and increases the risk of ear infections.

- Secondhand smoke exposure can cause children who already have asthma to experience more frequent and severe attacks.

Exposure of adults to secondhand smoke has immediate adverse effects on the cardiovascular system and causes coronary heart disease and lung cancer.

- Concentrations of many cancer-causing and toxic chemicals are higher in secondhand smoke than in the smoke inhaled by smokers.

- Breathing secondhand smoke for even a short time can have immediate adverse effects on the cardiovascular system and interferes with the normal functioning of the heart, blood, and vascular systems in ways that increase the risk of a heart attack.

- Nonsmokers who are exposed to secondhand smoke at home or at work increase their risk of developing heart disease by 25–30%.

- Nonsmokers who are exposed to secondhand smoke at home or at work increase their risk of developing lung cancer by 20–30%.

The scientific evidence indicates that there is no risk-free level of exposure to secondhand smoke.

- Short exposures to secondhand smoke can cause blood platelets to become stickier, damage the lining of blood vessels, decrease coronary flow velocity reserves, and reduce heart rate variability, potentially increasing the risk of a heart attack.

- Secondhand smoke contains many chemicals that can quickly irritate and damage the lining of the airways. Even brief exposure can result in upper airway changes in healthy persons and can lead to more frequent and more asthma attacks in children who already have asthma.

Eliminating smoking in indoor spaces fully protects nonsmokers from exposure to secondhand smoke. Separating smokers from nonsmokers, cleaning the air, and ventilating buildings cannot eliminate exposures of nonsmokers to secondhand smoke.

- Conventional air cleaning systems can remove large particles, but not the smaller particles or the gases found in secondhand smoke.

- Routine operation of a heating, ventilating, and air conditioning system can distribute secondhand smoke throughout a building.

- The American Society of Heating, Refrigerating and Air-Conditioning Engineers (ASHRAE), the preeminent U.S. body on ventilation issues, has concluded that ventilation technology cannot be relied on to control health risks from secondhand smoke exposure.

❖ It's A Fact!!

Inhaling secondhand smoke causes lung cancer in nonsmoking adults. Approximately 3,000 lung cancer deaths occur each year among adult nonsmokers in the United States as a result of exposure to secondhand smoke. The Surgeon General estimates that living with a smoker increases a nonsmoker's chances of developing lung cancer by 20 to 30%.

Some research suggests that secondhand smoke may increase the risk of breast cancer, nasal sinus cavity cancer, and nasopharyngeal cancer in adults, and leukemia, lymphoma, and brain tumors in children. Additional research is needed to learn whether a link exists between secondhand smoke exposure and these cancers.

Source: Excerpted from "Secondhand Smoke: Questions and Answers," National Cancer Institute, August 1, 2007.

There Is No Risk-Free Level Of Exposure To Secondhand Smoke

The U.S. Surgeon General has concluded that breathing even a little secondhand smoke poses a risk to your health.

- Scientific evidence indicates that there is no risk-free level of exposure to secondhand smoke.

- Breathing even a little secondhand smoke can be harmful to your health.

- Secondhand smoke causes lung cancer.

- Secondhand smoke is a known human carcinogen and contains more than 50 chemicals that can cause cancer.

- Concentrations of many cancer-causing and toxic chemicals are potentially higher in secondhand smoke than in the smoke inhaled by smokers.

Secondhand smoke causes heart disease.

- Breathing secondhand smoke for even a short time can have immediate adverse effects on the cardiovascular system, interfering with the normal functioning of the heart, blood, and vascular systems in ways that increase the risk of heart attack.

- Even a short time in a smoky room can cause your blood platelets to become stickier, damage the lining of blood vessels, decrease coronary flow velocity reserves, and reduce heart rate variability.

- Persons who already have heart disease are at especially high risk of suffering adverse affects from breathing secondhand smoke, and should take special precautions to avoid even brief exposure.

Secondhand smoke causes acute respiratory effects.

- Secondhand smoke contains many chemicals that can quickly irritate and damage the lining of the airways.

- Even brief exposure can trigger respiratory symptoms, including cough, phlegm, wheezing, and breathlessness.

- Brief exposure to secondhand smoke can trigger an asthma attack in children with asthma.

- Persons who already have asthma or other respiratory conditions are at especially high risk for being affected by secondhand smoke, and should take special precautions to avoid secondhand smoke exposure.

Secondhand smoke can cause sudden infant death syndrome (SIDS) and other health consequences in infants and children.

- Smoking by women during pregnancy has been known for some time to cause SIDS.

- Infants who are exposed to secondhand smoke after birth are also at greater risk of SIDS.

Children exposed to secondhand smoke are also at an increased risk for acute respiratory infections, ear problems, and more severe asthma. Smoking by parents causes respiratory symptoms and slows lung growth in their children.

Separating smokers from nonsmokers, cleaning the air, and ventilating buildings cannot eliminate secondhand smoke exposure. The American Society of Heating, Refrigerating and Air-Conditioning Engineers (ASHRAE), the preeminent U.S. standard-setting body on ventilation issues, has concluded that ventilation technology cannot be relied on to completely control health risks from secondhand smoke exposure. Conventional air cleaning systems can remove large particles, but not the smaller particles or the gases found in secondhand smoke. Operation of a heating, ventilating, and air conditioning system can distribute secondhand smoke throughout a building.

Secondhand Smoke Exposure In The Home

The home is the place where children are most exposed to secondhand smoke and a major location of secondhand smoke exposure for adults.

Children who live in homes where smoking is allowed have higher levels of cotinine (a biological marker of secondhand smoke exposure) than children who live in homes where smoking is not allowed. As the number of cigarettes smoked in the home increases, children's cotinine levels rise.

Although secondhand smoke exposure among children has declined over the past 15 years, children remain more heavily exposed to secondhand smoke than adults. Almost 60% of U.S. children aged 3–11 years—or almost 22 million children—are exposed to secondhand smoke. About 25% of children aged 3–11 years live with at least one smoker, as compared to only about 7% of nonsmoking adults.

Secondhand smoke exposure in the home has been consistently linked to a significant increase in both heart disease and lung cancer risk among adult nonsmokers.

♣ It's A Fact!!

There is no safe level of exposure to secondhand smoke. Studies have shown that even low levels of secondhand smoke exposure can be harmful. The only way to fully protect nonsmokers from secondhand smoke exposure is to completely eliminate smoking in indoor spaces. Separating smokers from nonsmokers, cleaning the air, and ventilating buildings cannot completely eliminate secondhand smoke exposure.

Source: Excerpted from "Secondhand Smoke: Questions and Answers," National Cancer Institute, August 1, 2007.

According to the Census Bureau's Current Population Survey, the proportion of households with smoke-free home rules increased from 43% in 1992–93 to 66% in 2001–02.

The proportion of persons who are covered by smoke-free home rules varies somewhat by region and state. For example, as of 2001–2002 this figure ranged from 51% in Kentucky to 86% in Utah among residents aged 15 years and older.

The Surgeon General has concluded that eliminating smoking in indoor spaces is the only way to fully protect nonsmokers from secondhand smoke exposure. Separating smokers from nonsmokers, cleaning the air, and ventilating buildings cannot completely eliminate secondhand smoke exposure.

Smoke-free rules in homes and vehicles can reduce secondhand smoke exposure among children and nonsmoking adults. Some studies indicate that these rules can also help smokers quit and can reduce the risk of adolescents becoming smokers.

Secondhand Smoke Is Toxic And Poisonous

The National Toxicology Program estimates that at least 250 chemicals in secondhand smoke are known to be toxic or carcinogenic (cancer causing).

Secondhand smoke contains a number of poisonous gases and chemicals, including hydrogen cyanide (used in chemical weapons), carbon monoxide (found in car exhaust), butane (used in lighter fluid), ammonia (used in household cleaners), and toluene (found in paint thinners). Some of the toxic metals contained in secondhand smoke include arsenic (used in pesticides), lead (formerly found in paint), chromium (used to make steel), and cadmium (used to make batteries). There are more than 50 cancer-causing chemicals in secondhand smoke that fall into different chemical classes, including:

- Polynuclear aromatic hydrocarbons (PAHs) (such as benzo[a]pyrene);

  N-Nitrosamines (such as tobacco-specific nitrosamines);

- Aromatic amines (such as 4-aminobiphenyl);

- Aldehydes (such as formaldehyde);

- Miscellaneous organic chemicals (such as benzene and vinyl chloride); and

- Inorganic compounds (such as those containing metals like arsenic, beryllium, cadmium, lead, nickel and radioactive polonium-210).

Eleven compounds in tobacco smoke (2-naphthylamine, 4-aminobiphenyl, benzene, vinyl chloride, ethylene oxide, arsenic, beryllium, nickel compounds, chromium, cadmium and polonium-210) have been identified by the International Agency for Research on Cancer as Group 1 (known human carcinogen) carcinogens.

Secondhand smoke has been designated as a known human carcinogen (cancer-causing agent) by the U.S. Environmental Protection Agency, National Toxicology Program and the International Agency for Research on Cancer (IARC). The National Institute for Occupational Safety and Health has concluded that secondhand smoke is an occupational carcinogen.

Secondhand smoke is composed of sidestream smoke (the smoke released from the burning end of a cigarette) and exhaled mainstream smoke (the smoke exhaled by the smoker). Because sidestream smoke is generated at lower temperatures and under different conditions than mainstream smoke, it contains higher concentrations of many of the toxins found in inhaled cigarette smoke.

♣ It's A Fact!!

Many state and local governments have passed laws prohibiting smoking in public facilities such as schools, hospitals, airports, and bus terminals. Increasingly, state and local governments are also requiring private workplaces, including restaurants and bars, to be smoke free. To highlight the significant risk from secondhand smoke exposure, the National Cancer Institute, a component of the National Institutes of Health, holds meetings and conferences in states, counties, cities, or towns that are smoke free, unless certain circumstances justify an exception to this policy.

Source: Excerpted from "Secondhand Smoke: Questions and Answers," National Cancer Institute, August 1, 2007.

Part Three

Cancers Associated With Tobacco Use

Chapter 22

Questions And Answers About Smoking And Cancer

How does smoking affect my risk for cancer?

Certain agents in tobacco smoke can damage important genes that control the growth of cells, which increases a person's risk for many types of cancer.

Lung cancer is the leading cause of cancer death. About 87% of lung cancer cases are caused by smoking. Smokers are about 20 times more likely to develop lung cancer than nonsmokers. Smoking also causes cancers of the mouth, throat, larynx (voice box), and esophagus, and it increases a person's risk of developing cancer of the pancreas, kidney, bladder, cervix, and stomach. Smoking may also contribute to the development of acute myeloid leukemia, which is a cancer of the blood.

For smoking-attributable cancers, the risk generally increases with the number of cigarettes smoked and the number of years of smoking. Risks generally decrease after a person quits completely. Ten years after quitting, the risk of developing lung cancer decreases by as much as half.

About This Chapter: This chapter begins with an excerpt from "Smoking and Tobacco Use: Frequently Asked Questions," Centers for Disease Control and Prevention (CDC), 2006. It continues with excerpts from "Quitting Smoking: Why to Quit and how to Get Help," National Cancer Institute, August 17, 2007.

✤ It's A Fact!!
Understanding Cancer

Cancer is a group of many related diseases. All cancers begin in cells, the body's basic unit of life. Cells make up tissues, and tissues make up the organs of the body.

Normally, cells grow and divide to form new cells as the body needs them. When cells grow old and die, new cells take their place.

Sometimes this orderly process goes wrong. New cells form when the body does not need them, and old cells do not die when they should. These extra cells can form a mass of tissue called a growth or tumor.

Tumors can be benign or malignant:

- **Benign Tumors:** Benign tumors are not cancer. Usually, doctors can remove them. Cells from benign tumors do not spread to other parts of the body. In most cases, benign tumors do not come back after they are removed. Most important, benign tumors are rarely a threat to life.

- **Malignant Tumors:** Malignant tumors are cancer. They are generally more serious. Cancer cells can invade and damage nearby tissues and organs. Also, cancer cells can break away from a malignant tumor and enter the bloodstream or the lymphatic system. That is how cancer cells spread from the original (primary) tumor to form new tumors in other organs. The spread of cancer is called metastasis.

Source: Excerpted from "What You Need to Know about Bladder Cancer," National Cancer Institute, September 16, 2002.

What parts of the body are harmed by smoking?

Smoking harms nearly every organ of the body and diminishes a person's overall health. Smoking is a leading cause of cancer and of death from cancer. It causes cancers of the lung, esophagus, larynx (voice box), mouth, throat, kidney, bladder, pancreas, stomach, and cervix, as well as acute myeloid leukemia.

Smoking also causes heart disease, stroke, lung disease (chronic bronchitis and emphysema), hip fractures, and cataracts. Smokers are at higher risk of developing pneumonia and other airway infections.

A pregnant smoker is at higher risk of having her baby born too early and with an abnormally low weight. A woman who smokes during or after pregnancy increases her infant's risk of death from sudden infant death syndrome (SIDS).

Millions of Americans have health problems caused by smoking. Cigarette smoking and exposure to tobacco smoke cause an estimated average of 438,000 premature deaths each year in the United States. Of these premature deaths, about 40% are from cancer, 35% are from heart disease and stroke, and 25% are from lung disease. Smoking is the leading cause of premature, preventable death in this country.

Regardless of their age, smokers can substantially reduce their risk of disease, including cancer, by quitting.

What chemicals in tobacco smoke cause cancer?

Tobacco smoke contains chemicals that are harmful to both smokers and nonsmokers. Breathing even a little tobacco smoke can be harmful. Of the 4,000 chemicals in tobacco smoke, at least 250 are known to be harmful. The toxic chemicals found in smoke include hydrogen cyanide (used in chemical weapons), carbon monoxide (found in car exhaust), formaldehyde (used as an embalming fluid), ammonia (used in household cleaners), and toluene (found in paint thinners).

Of the 250 known harmful chemicals in tobacco smoke, more than 50 have been found to cause cancer. These chemicals include the following:

- arsenic (a heavy metal toxin)
- benzene (a chemical found in gasoline)
- beryllium (a toxic metal)
- cadmium (a metal used in batteries)
- chromium (a metallic element)
- ethylene oxide (a chemical used to sterilize medical devices)
- nickel (a metallic element)
- polonium-210 (a chemical element that gives off radiation)
- vinyl chloride (a toxic substance used in plastics manufacture)

What are the benefits of quitting smoking?

The immediate health benefits of quitting smoking are substantial. Heart rate and blood pressure, which were abnormally high while smoking, begin to return to normal. Within a few hours, the level of carbon monoxide in the blood begins to decline. (Carbon monoxide, a colorless, odorless gas found in cigarette smoke, reduces the blood's ability to carry oxygen.) Within a few weeks, people who quit smoking have improved circulation, don't produce as much phlegm, and don't cough or wheeze as often. Within several months of quitting, people can expect significant improvements in lung function.

Quitting smoking also reduces the risk of cancer and other diseases, such as heart disease and lung disease, caused by smoking. People who quit smoking, regardless of their age, are less likely than those who continue to smoke to die from smoking-related illness. Studies have shown that quitting at about age 30 reduces the chance of dying from smoking-related diseases by more than 90%. People who quit at about age 50 reduce their risk of dying prematurely by 50% compared with those who continue to smoke. Even people who quit at about age 60 or older live longer than those who continue to smoke.

♣ It's A Fact!!
Tobacco and Cancer

Tobacco is one of the strongest cancer-causing agents. Tobacco use is associated with a number of different cancers, including lung cancer, as well as with chronic lung diseases and cardiovascular diseases.

- Lung cancer is the leading cause of cancer death among both men and women in the United States, with 90% of lung cancer deaths among men and approximately 80% of lung cancer deaths among women attributed to smoking.

- Smoking also increases the risk of many other types of cancer, including cancers of the throat, mouth, pancreas, kidney, bladder, and cervix.

Source: Excerpted from "Smoking," National Cancer Institute, an undated fact sheet available at http://www.cancer.gov/cancertopics/smoking. Accessed December 28, 2009.

Does quitting smoking lower the risk of cancer?

Quitting smoking substantially reduces the risk of developing and dying from cancer, and this benefit increases the longer a person remains smoke free. However, even after many years of not smoking, the risk of lung cancer in former smokers remains higher than in people who have never smoked.

The risk of premature death and the chance of developing cancer due to cigarettes depend on the number of years of smoking, the number of cigarettes smoked per day, the age at which smoking began, and the presence or absence of illness at the time of quitting. For people who have already developed cancer, quitting smoking reduces the risk of developing a second cancer.

Should someone already diagnosed with cancer bother to quit smoking?

Yes. There are many reasons that people diagnosed with cancer should quit smoking. For those having surgery or other treatments, quitting smoking helps improve the body's ability to heal and respond to the cancer treatment, and it lowers the risk of pneumonia and respiratory failure. Also, quitting smoking may lower the risk of the cancer returning or a second cancer forming.

Chapter 23

Bladder Cancer

The Bladder And Cancer

The bladder is a hollow organ in the lower abdomen. It stores urine, the liquid waste produced by the kidneys. Urine passes from each kidney into the bladder through a tube called a ureter.

An outer layer of muscle surrounds the inner lining of the bladder. When the bladder is full, the muscles in the bladder wall can tighten to allow urination. Urine leaves the bladder through another tube, the urethra.

There are three types of bladder cancer that begin in cells in the lining of the bladder. Cancer that is only in cells in the lining of the bladder is called superficial bladder cancer. The doctor might call it carcinoma in situ. This type of bladder cancer often comes back after treatment. If this happens, the disease most often recurs as another superficial cancer in the bladder.

Cancer that begins as a superficial tumor may grow through the lining and into the muscular wall of the bladder. This is known as invasive cancer. Invasive cancer may extend through the bladder wall. It may grow into a nearby organ such as the uterus or vagina (in women) or the prostate gland (in men). It also may invade the wall of the abdomen.

About This Chapter: Text in this chapter is excerpted from "What You Need to Know about Bladder Cancer," National Cancer Institute, September 16, 2002.

✎ **What's It Mean?**

The three types of bladder cancer that begin in cells in the lining of the bladder are named for the type of cells that become malignant:

Transitional Cell Carcinoma: Cancer that begins in cells in the innermost tissue layer of the bladder. These cells are able to stretch when the bladder is full and shrink when it is emptied. Most bladder cancers begin in transitional cells.

Squamous Cell Carcinoma: Cancer that begins in squamous cells, which are thin, flat cells that may form in the bladder after a long- term infection or irritation.

Adenocarcinoma: Cancer that begins in glandular (secretory) cells that may form in the bladder after a long-term inflammation or irritation.

When bladder cancer spreads outside the bladder, cancer cells are often found in nearby lymph nodes. If the cancer has reached these nodes, cancer cells may have spread to other lymph nodes or other organs, such as the lungs, liver, or bones.

When cancer spreads (metastasizes) from its original place to another part of the body, the new tumor has the same kind of abnormal cells and the same name as the primary tumor. For example, if bladder cancer spreads to the lungs, the cancer cells in the lungs are actually bladder cancer cells. The disease is metastatic bladder cancer, not lung cancer. It is treated as bladder cancer, not as lung cancer. Doctors sometimes call the new tumor "distant" disease.

Who's At Risk For Bladder Cancer?

No one knows the exact causes of bladder cancer. However, it is clear that this disease is not contagious. No one can "catch" cancer from another person.

People who get bladder cancer are more likely than other people to have certain risk factors. A risk factor is something that increases a person's chance of developing the disease.

Still, most people with known risk factors do not get bladder cancer, and many who do get this disease have none of these factors. Doctors can seldom explain why one person gets this cancer and another does not.

Studies have found the following risk factors for bladder cancer:

- **Age:** The chance of getting bladder cancer goes up as people get older.

- **Tobacco:** The use of tobacco is a major risk factor. Cigarette smokers are two to three times more likely than nonsmokers to get bladder cancer. Pipe and cigar smokers are also at increased risk.

- **Occupation:** Some workers have a higher risk of getting bladder cancer because of carcinogens in the workplace. Workers in the rubber, chemical, and leather industries are at risk. So are hairdressers, machinists, metal workers, printers, painters, textile workers, and truck drivers.

- **Infections:** Being infected with certain parasites increases the risk of bladder cancer. These parasites are common in tropical areas but not in the United States.

- **Cyclophosphamide Or Arsenic:** These drugs are used to treat cancer and some other conditions. They raise the risk of bladder cancer.

- **Race:** Whites get bladder cancer twice as often as African Americans and Hispanics. The lowest rates are among Asians.

- **Gender:** Men are two to three times more likely than women to get bladder cancer.

- **Family History:** People with family members who have bladder cancer are more likely to get the disease.

- **Personal History:** People who have had bladder cancer have an increased chance of getting the disease again.

♣ It's A Fact!!
Tobacco Use And Bladder Cancer

Tobacco use is a major risk factor for bladder cancer. When compared with nonsmokers, cigarette smokers are two to three times more likely to get bladder cancer. Pipe and cigar smokers are also at increased risk.

Symptoms

Common symptoms of bladder cancer include blood in the urine (making the urine slightly rusty to deep red), pain during urination, and frequent urination, or feeling the need to urinate without results.

These symptoms are not sure signs of bladder cancer. Infections, benign tumors, bladder stones, or other problems also can cause these symptoms. Anyone with these symptoms should see a doctor so that the doctor can diagnose and treat any problem as early as possible. People with symptoms like these may see their family doctor or a urologist, a doctor who specializes in diseases of the urinary system.

Diagnosis

If a patient has symptoms that suggest bladder cancer, the doctor may check general signs of health and may order lab tests. The person may have one or more of the following procedures:

- **Physical Exam:** The doctor feels the abdomen and pelvis for tumors. The physical exam may include a rectal or vaginal exam.

- **Urine Tests:** The laboratory checks the urine for blood, cancer cells, and other signs of disease.

- **Intravenous Pyelogram:** The doctor injects dye into a blood vessel. The dye collects in the urine, making the bladder show up on x-rays.

- **Cystoscopy:** The doctor uses a thin, lighted tube (cystoscope) to look directly into the bladder. The doctor inserts the cystoscope into the bladder through the urethra to examine the lining of the bladder. The patient may need anesthesia for this procedure.

- **Biopsy:** The doctor can remove samples of tissue with the cystoscope. A pathologist then examines the tissue under a microscope. The removal of tissue to look for cancer cells is called a biopsy. In many cases, a biopsy is the only sure way to tell whether cancer is present. For a small number of patients, the doctor removes the entire cancerous area during the biopsy. For these patients, bladder cancer is diagnosed and treated in a single procedure.

Staging

If bladder cancer is diagnosed, the doctor needs to know the stage, or extent, of the disease to plan the best treatment. Staging is a careful attempt to find out whether the cancer has invaded the bladder wall, whether the disease has spread, and if so, to what parts of the body.

The doctor may determine the stage of bladder cancer at the time of diagnosis, or may need to give the patient more tests. Such tests may include imaging tests—CT scan, magnetic resonance imaging (MRI), sonogram, intravenous pyelogram, bone scan, or chest x-ray. Sometimes staging is not complete until the patient has surgery.

Methods Of Treatment

People with bladder cancer have many treatment options. They may have surgery, radiation therapy, chemotherapy, or biological therapy. Some patients get a combination of therapies. Clinical trials are also an important option for people with all stages of bladder cancer.

♣ It's A Fact!!
Uncertain Risks

Chlorine is added to water to make it safe to drink. It kills deadly bacteria. However, chlorine by-products sometimes can form in chlorinated water. Researchers have been studying chlorine by-products for more than 25 years. So far, there is no proof that chlorinated water causes bladder cancer in people. Studies continue to look at this question.

Some studies have found that saccharin, an artificial sweetener, causes bladder cancer in animals. However, research does not show that saccharin causes cancer in people.

Surgery

Surgery is a common treatment for bladder cancer. The type of surgery depends largely on the stage and grade of the tumor.

- **Transurethral Resection:** The doctor may treat early (superficial) bladder cancer with transurethral resection (TUR). During TUR, the doctor inserts a cystoscope into the bladder through the urethra. The doctor then uses a tool with a small wire loop on the end to remove the cancer and to burn away any remaining cancer cells with an electric current. (This is called fulguration.) The patient may need to be in the hospital and may need anesthesia. After TUR, patients may also have chemotherapy or biological therapy.

- **Radical Cystectomy:** For invasive bladder cancer, the most common type of surgery is radical cystectomy. The doctor also chooses this type of surgery when superficial cancer involves a large part of the bladder. Radical cystectomy is the removal of the entire bladder, the nearby lymph nodes, part of the urethra, and the nearby organs that may contain cancer cells. In men, the nearby organs that are removed are the prostate, seminal vesicles, and part of the vas deferens. In women, the uterus, ovaries, fallopian tubes, and part of the vagina are removed.

- **Segmental Cystectomy:** In some cases, the doctor may remove only part of the bladder in a procedure called segmental cystectomy. The doctor chooses this type of surgery when a patient has a low-grade cancer that has invaded the bladder wall in just one area.

Sometimes, when the cancer has spread outside the bladder and cannot be completely removed, the surgeon removes the bladder but does not try to get rid of all the cancer. Or, the surgeon does not remove the bladder but makes another way for urine to leave the body. The goal of the surgery may be to relieve urinary blockage or other symptoms caused by the cancer.

When the entire bladder is removed, the surgeon makes another way to collect urine. The patient may wear a bag outside the body, or the surgeon may create a pouch inside the body with part of the intestine.

Radiation Therapy And Chemotherapy

Radiation therapy (also called radiotherapy) uses high-energy rays to kill cancer cells. Like surgery, radiation therapy is local therapy. It affects cancer cells only in the treated area. A small number of patients may have radiation therapy before surgery to shrink the tumor. Others may have it after surgery to kill cancer cells that may remain in the area. Sometimes, patients who cannot have surgery have radiation therapy instead.

Chemotherapy uses drugs to kill cancer cells. The doctor may use one drug or a combination of drugs.

For patients with superficial bladder cancer, the doctor may use intravesical chemotherapy after removing the cancer with TUR. This is local therapy. The doctor inserts a tube (catheter) through the urethra and puts liquid drugs in the bladder through the catheter. The drugs remain in the bladder for several hours. They mainly affect the cells in the bladder. Usually, the patient has this treatment once a week for several weeks. Sometimes, the treatments continue once or several times a month for up to a year.

If the cancer has deeply invaded the bladder or spread to lymph nodes or other organs, the doctor may give drugs through a vein. This treatment is called intravenous chemotherapy. It is systemic therapy, meaning that the drugs flow through the bloodstream to nearly every part of the body. The drugs are usually given in cycles so that a recovery period follows every treatment period.

Other Treatments

Biological therapy (also called immunotherapy) uses the body's natural ability (immune system) to fight cancer. Biological therapy is most often used after TUR for superficial bladder cancer. This helps prevent the cancer from coming back.

The doctor may use intravesical biological therapy with BCG solution. BCG solution contains live, weakened bacteria. The bacteria stimulate the immune system to kill cancer cells in the bladder. The doctor uses a catheter to put the solution in the bladder. The patient must hold the solution in the bladder for about two hours. BCG treatment is usually done once a week for six weeks.

Side Effects Of Cancer Treatment

Because cancer treatment may damage healthy cells and tissues, unwanted side effects sometimes occur. These side effects depend on many factors, including the type and extent of the treatment. Side effects may not be the same for each person, and they may even change from one treatment session to the next. Doctors and nurses will explain the possible side effects of treatment and how they will help the patient manage them.

Surgery Side Effects

For a few days after TUR, patients may have some blood in their urine and difficulty or pain when urinating. Otherwise, TUR generally causes few problems.

After cystectomy, most patients are uncomfortable during the first few days. However, medicine can control the pain. Also, it is common to feel tired or weak for a while.

After segmental cystectomy, patients may not be able to hold as much urine in their bladder as they used to, and they may need to urinate more often. In most cases, this problem is temporary, but some patients may have long-lasting changes in how much urine they can hold.

If the surgeon removes the bladder, the patient needs a new way to store and pass urine. In one common method, the surgeon uses a piece of the person's small intestine to form a new tube through which urine can pass. The surgeon attaches one end of the tube to the ureters and connects the other end to a new opening in the wall of the abdomen. This opening is called a stoma. A flat bag fits over the stoma to collect urine, and a special adhesive holds it in place. The operation to create the stoma is called a urostomy or an ostomy.

For some patients, the doctor is able to use a part of the small intestine to make a storage pouch (called a continent reservoir) inside the body. Urine collects in the pouch instead of going into a bag. The surgeon connects the pouch to the urethra or to a stoma. If the surgeon connects the pouch to a stoma, the patient uses a catheter to drain the urine.

Bladder cancer surgery may affect a person's sexual function. Because the surgeon removes the uterus and ovaries in a radical cystectomy, women are not able to get pregnant. Also, menopause occurs at once. Hot flashes and other symptoms of menopause caused by surgery may be more severe than those caused by natural menopause. If the surgeon removes part of the vagina during a radical cystectomy, sexual intercourse may be difficult.

In the past, nearly all men were impotent after radical cystectomy, but improvements in surgery have made it possible for some men to avoid this problem. Men who have had their prostate gland and seminal vesicles removed no longer produce semen, so they have dry orgasms. Men who wish to father children may consider sperm banking before surgery or sperm retrieval later on.

It is natural for a patient to worry about the effects of bladder cancer surgery on sexuality. Patients may want to talk with the doctor about possible side effects and how long these side effects are likely to last. Whatever the outlook, it may be helpful for patients and their partners to talk about their feelings and help one another find ways to share intimacy during and after treatment.

Radiation Therapy Side Effects

The side effects of radiation therapy depend mainly on the treatment dose and the part of the body that is treated. Patients are likely to become very tired during radiation therapy, especially in the later weeks of treatment. Resting is important, but doctors usually advise patients to try to stay as active as they can.

External radiation may permanently darken or "bronze" the skin in the treated area. Patients commonly lose hair in the treated area and their skin may become red, dry, tender, and itchy. These problems are temporary, and the doctor can suggest ways to relieve them.

❖ It's A Fact!!

Each year in the United States, bladder cancer is diagnosed in 38,000 men and 15,000 women. It is the fourth most common type of cancer in men and the eighth most common in women.

Radiation therapy to the abdomen may cause nausea, vomiting, diarrhea, or urinary discomfort. The doctor can suggest medicines to ease these problems.

Radiation therapy also may cause a decrease in the number of white blood cells, cells that help protect the body against infection. If the blood counts are low, the doctor or nurse may suggest ways to avoid getting an infection. Also, the patient may not get more radiation therapy until blood counts improve. The doctor will check the patient's blood counts regularly and change the treatment schedule if it is necessary.

For both men and women, radiation treatment for bladder cancer can affect sexuality. Women may experience vaginal dryness, and men may have difficulty with erections.

Chemotherapy Side Effects

The side effects of chemotherapy depend mainly on the drugs and the doses the patient receives as well as how the drugs are given. In addition, as with other types of treatment, side effects vary from patient to patient.

Anticancer drugs that are placed in the bladder cause irritation, with some discomfort or bleeding that lasts for a few days after treatment. Some drugs may cause a rash when they come into contact with the skin or genitals.

Systemic chemotherapy affects rapidly dividing cells throughout the body, including blood cells. Blood cells fight infection, help the blood to clot, and carry oxygen to all parts of the body. When anticancer drugs damage blood cells, patients are more likely to get infections, may bruise or bleed easily, and may have less energy. Cells in hair roots and cells that line the digestive tract also divide rapidly. As a result, patients may lose their hair and may have other side effects such as poor appetite, nausea and vomiting, or mouth sores. Usually, these side effects go away gradually during the recovery periods between treatments or after treatment is over.

Certain drugs used in the treatment of bladder cancer also may cause kidney damage. To protect the kidneys, patients need a lot of fluid. The nurse may give the patient fluids by vein before and after treatment. Also, the patient may need to drink a lot of fluids during treatment with these drugs.

Biological Therapy Side Effects

BCG therapy can irritate the bladder. Patients may feel an urgent need to urinate, and may need to urinate frequently. Patients also may have pain, especially when urinating. They may feel tired. Some patients may have blood in their urine, nausea, a low-grade fever, or chills.

Follow-Up Care

Follow-up care after treatment for bladder cancer is important. Bladder cancer can return in the bladder or elsewhere in the body. Therefore, people who have had bladder cancer may wish to discuss the chance of recurrence with the doctor.

Chapter 24

Cervical Cancer

The Cervix

The cervix is part of a woman's reproductive system. It's in the pelvis. The cervix is the lower, narrow part of the uterus (womb). The cervix is a passageway that serves the following functions:

- It connects the uterus to the vagina. During a menstrual period, blood flows from the uterus through the cervix into the vagina. The vagina leads to the outside of the body.

- It makes mucus. During sex, mucus helps sperm move from the vagina through the cervix into the uterus.

- It is tightly closed during pregnancy to help keep the baby inside the uterus. During childbirth, the cervix opens to allow the baby to pass through the vagina.

Growths on the cervix can be benign or malignant. Benign growths are not cancer. They are not as harmful as malignant growths (cancer). Benign growths (polyps, cysts, or genital warts) are rarely a threat to life. They don't invade the tissues around them. Malignant growths (cervical cancer) may sometimes be a threat to life. They can invade nearby tissues and organs and can spread to other parts of the body.

About This Chapter: Text in this chapter is excerpted from "What You Need to Know about Cancer of the Cervix," National Cancer Institute, November 20, 2008.

> ### ✎ What's It Mean?
>
> HPV Infection: HPV (human papillomavirus) is a group of viruses that can infect the cervix. An HPV infection that doesn't go away can cause cervical cancer in some women. HPV is the cause of nearly all cervical cancers.
>
> Source: National Cancer Institute, 2008.

Cervical cancer begins in cells on the surface of the cervix. Over time, the cervical cancer can invade more deeply into the cervix and nearby tissues. The cancer cells can spread by breaking away from the original (primary) tumor. They enter blood vessels or lymph vessels, which branch into all the tissues of the body. The cancer cells may attach to other tissues and grow to form new tumors that may damage those tissues. The spread of cancer is called metastasis.

Risk Factors

Doctors cannot always explain why one woman develops cervical cancer and another does not. However, we do know that a woman with certain risk factors may be more likely than others to develop cervical cancer. A risk factor is something that may increase the chance of developing a disease.

Studies have found a number of factors that may increase the risk of cervical cancer. For example, infection with HPV (human papillomavirus) is the main cause of cervical cancer.

HPV infections are very common. These viruses are passed from person to person through sexual contact. Most adults have been infected with HPV at some time in their lives, but most infections clear up on their own.

Some types of HPV can cause changes to cells in the cervix. If these changes are found early, cervical cancer can be prevented by removing or killing the changed cells before they can become cancer cells.

A vaccine for females ages nine to 26 protects against two types of HPV infection that cause cervical cancer.

HPV infection and other risk factors may act together to increase the risk even more:

- **Lack Of Regular Pap Tests:** Cervical cancer is more common among women who don't have regular Pap tests. The Pap test helps doctors find abnormal cells. Removing or killing the abnormal cells usually prevents cervical cancer.

- **Smoking:** Among women who are infected with HPV, smoking cigarettes slightly increases the risk of cervical cancer.

- **Weakened Immune System:** Infection with HIV (the virus that causes AIDS) or taking drugs that suppress the immune system increases the risk of cervical cancer.

- **Sexual History:** Women who have had many sexual partners have a higher risk of developing cervical cancer. Also, a woman who has had sex with a man who has had many sexual partners may be at higher risk of developing cervical cancer. In both cases, the risk of developing cervical cancer is higher because these women have a higher risk of HPV infection.

- **Using Birth Control Pills For A Long Time:** Using birth control pills for a long time (five or more years) may slightly increase the risk of cervical cancer among women with HPV infection. However, the risk decreases quickly when women stop using birth control pills.

- **Having Many Children:** Studies suggest that giving birth to many children (five or more) may slightly increase the risk of cervical cancer among women with HPV infection.

✔ Quick Tip

If you smoke, you should be screened for any smoking-related disorders. Have your cholesterol and blood pressure checked regularly. Women should have annual Pap smears to detect cervical cancer.

Source: Excerpted from "Smoking," © 2010 A.D.A.M, Inc. Reprinted with permission.

- **DES (Diethylstilbestrol):** DES may increase the risk of a rare form of cervical cancer in daughters exposed to this drug before birth. DES was given to some pregnant women in the United States between about 1940 and 1971. (It is no longer given to pregnant women.)

Having an HPV infection or other risk factors does not mean that a woman will develop cervical cancer. Most women who have risk factors for cervical cancer never develop it.

Symptoms

Early cervical cancers usually don't cause symptoms. When the cancer grows larger, women may notice one or more of these symptoms:

- Abnormal vaginal bleeding
- Bleeding that occurs between regular menstrual periods
- Bleeding after sexual intercourse, douching, or a pelvic exam
- Menstrual periods that last longer and are heavier than before
- Bleeding after going through menopause
- Increased vaginal discharge
- Pelvic pain
- Pain during sex

Infections or other health problems may also cause these symptoms. Only a doctor can tell for sure. A woman with any of these symptoms should tell her doctor so that problems can be diagnosed and treated as early as possible.

✤ It's A Fact!!

Research shows that people with cancer feel better when they stay active. Walking, yoga, swimming, and other activities can keep you strong and increase your energy. Exercise may reduce nausea and pain and make treatment easier to handle. It also can help relieve stress. Whatever physical activity you choose, be sure to talk to your doctor before you start. Also, if your activity causes you pain or other problems, be sure to let your doctor or nurse know about it.

Source: National Cancer Institute, 2008.

Detection And Diagnosis

Doctors recommend that women help reduce their risk of cervical cancer by having regular Pap tests. A Pap test (sometimes called Pap smear or cervical smear) is a simple test used to look at cervical cells. Pap tests can find cervical cancer or abnormal cells that can lead to cervical cancer.

Finding and treating abnormal cells can prevent most cervical cancer. Also, the Pap test can help find cancer early, when treatment is more likely to be effective.

For most women, the Pap test is not painful. It's done in a doctor's office or clinic during a pelvic exam. The doctor or nurse scrapes a sample of cells from the cervix. A lab checks the cells under a microscope for cell changes. Most often, abnormal cells found by a Pap test are not cancerous. The same sample of cells may be tested for HPV infection.

If you have abnormal Pap or HPV test results, your doctor will suggest other tests to make a diagnosis:

- **Colposcopy:** The doctor uses a colposcope to look at the cervix. The colposcope combines a bright light with a magnifying lens to make tissue easier to see. It is not inserted into the vagina. A colposcopy is usually done in the doctor's office or clinic.

- **Biopsy:** Most women have tissue removed in the doctor's office with local anesthesia. A pathologist checks the tissue under a microscope for abnormal cells.

- **Punch Biopsy:** The doctor uses a sharp tool to pinch off small samples of cervical tissue.

- **LEEP:** The doctor uses an electric wire loop to slice off a thin, round piece of cervical tissue.

- **Endocervical Curettage:** The doctor uses a curette (a small, spoon-shaped instrument) to scrape a small sample of tissue from the cervix. Some doctors may use a thin, soft brush instead of a curette.

- **Conization:** The doctor removes a cone-shaped sample of tissue. A conization, or cone biopsy, lets the pathologist see if abnormal cells are in the tissue beneath the surface of the cervix. The doctor may do this test in the hospital under general anesthesia.

Removing tissue from the cervix may cause some bleeding or other discharge. The area usually heals quickly. Some women also feel some pain similar to menstrual cramps. Your doctor can suggest medicine that will help relieve your pain.

Staging

Staging is a careful attempt to find out whether the tumor has invaded nearby tissues, whether the cancer has spread and, if so, to what parts of the body. Cervical cancer spreads most often to nearby tissues in the pelvis, lymph nodes, or the lungs. It may also spread to the liver or bones.

When cancer spreads from its original place to another part of the body, the new tumor has the same kind of cancer cells and the same name as the original tumor. For example, if cervical cancer spreads to the lungs, the cancer cells in the lungs are actually cervical cancer cells. The disease is metastatic cervical cancer, not lung cancer. For that reason, it's treated as cervical cancer, not lung cancer. Doctors call the new tumor "distant" or metastatic disease.

Your doctor will do a pelvic exam, feel for swollen lymph nodes, and may remove additional tissue.

Treatment

Women with cervical cancer have many treatment options. The options are surgery, radiation therapy, chemotherapy, or a combination of methods.

The choice of treatment depends mainly on the size of the tumor and whether the cancer has spread. The treatment choice may also depend on whether you would like to become pregnant someday.

Your doctor may refer you to a specialist, or you may ask for a referral. You may want to see a gynecologic oncologist, a surgeon who specializes in treating female cancers. Other specialists who treat cervical cancer include gynecologists, medical oncologists, and radiation oncologists. Your health care team may also include an oncology nurse and a registered dietitian.

You may want to talk to your doctor about taking part in a clinical trial, a research study of new treatment methods.

Surgery

Surgery is an option for women with Stage I or II cervical cancer. The surgeon removes tissue that may contain cancer cells:

- **Radical Trachelectomy:** The surgeon removes the cervix, part of the vagina, and the lymph nodes in the pelvis. This option is for a small number of women with small tumors who want to try to get pregnant later on.
- **Total Hysterectomy:** The surgeon removes the cervix and uterus.
- **Radical Hysterectomy:** The surgeon removes the cervix, some tissue around the cervix, the uterus, and part of the vagina.

With either total or radical hysterectomy, the surgeon may remove other tissues:

- **Fallopian Tubes And Ovaries:** The surgeon may remove both fallopian tubes and ovaries. This surgery is called a salpingo-oophorectomy.
- **Lymph Nodes:** The surgeon may remove the lymph nodes near the tumor to see if they contain cancer. If cancer cells have reached the lymph nodes, it means the disease may have spread to other parts of the body.

Radiation Therapy

Radiation therapy (also called radiotherapy) is an option for women with any stage of cervical cancer. Women with early stage cervical cancer may choose radiation therapy instead of surgery. It also may be used after surgery to destroy any cancer cells that remain in the area. Women with cancer that extends beyond the cervix may have radiation therapy and chemotherapy.

Radiation therapy uses high-energy rays to kill cancer cells. It affects cells only in the treated area.

You may have dryness, itching, or burning in your vagina. Your doctor may advise you to wait to have sex until a few weeks after radiation treatment ends.

You are likely to become tired during radiation therapy, especially in the later weeks of treatment. Resting is important, but doctors usually advise patients to try to stay as active as they can.

Although the side effects of radiation therapy can be upsetting, they can usually be treated or controlled. Talk with your doctor or nurse about ways to relieve discomfort.

It may also help to know that most side effects go away when treatment ends. However, you may wish to discuss with your doctor the possible long-term effects of radiation therapy. For example, the radiation may make the vagina narrower. A narrow vagina can make sex or follow-up exams difficult. There are ways to prevent this problem. If it does occur, however, your health care team can tell you about ways to expand the vagina.

Another long-term effect is that radiation aimed at the pelvic area can harm the ovaries. Menstrual periods usually stop, and women may have hot flashes and vaginal dryness. Menstrual periods are more likely to return for younger women. Women who may want to get pregnant after radiation therapy should ask their health care team about ways to preserve their eggs before treatment starts.

✤ It's A Fact!!
Cancer Research

Doctors all over the country are conducting many types of clinical trials (research studies in which people volunteer to take part). They are studying new ways to treat cervical cancer. Some are also studying therapies that may improve the quality of life for women during or after cancer treatment.

Clinical trials are designed to answer important questions and to find out whether new approaches are safe and effective. Research already has led to advances in the prevention, diagnosis, and treatment of cervical cancer. Doctors continue to search for new and better ways to treat cervical cancer.

Source: National Cancer Institute, 2008.

Chemotherapy

For the treatment of cervical cancer, chemotherapy is usually combined with radiation therapy. For cancer that has spread to distant organs, chemotherapy alone may be used.

Chemotherapy uses drugs to kill cancer cells. The drugs for cervical cancer are usually given through a vein (intravenous). You may receive chemotherapy in a clinic, at the doctor's office, or at home. Some women need to stay in the hospital during treatment.

The side effects depend mainly on which drugs are given and how much. Chemotherapy kills fast-growing cancer cells, but the drugs can also harm normal cells that divide rapidly:

- **Blood Cells:** When chemotherapy lowers the levels of healthy blood cells, you're more likely to get infections, bruise or bleed easily, and feel very weak and tired.

- **Cells In Hair Roots:** Chemotherapy may cause hair loss. If you lose your hair, it will grow back, but it may change in color and texture.

- **Cells That Line The Digestive Tract:** Chemotherapy can cause a poor appetite, nausea and vomiting, diarrhea, or mouth and lip sores.

Other side effects include skin rash, tingling or numbness in your hands and feet, hearing problems, loss of balance, joint pain, or swollen legs and feet. Your health care team can suggest ways to control many of these problems. Most go away when treatment ends.

Follow-Up Care

You'll need regular checkups after treatment for cervical cancer. Checkups help ensure that any changes in your health are noted and treated if needed. If you have any health problems between checkups, you should contact your doctor.

Your doctor will check for the return of cancer. Even when the cancer seems to have been completely removed or destroyed, the disease sometimes returns because undetected cancer cells remained somewhere in the body after treatment. Checkups may include a physical exam, Pap tests, and chest x-rays.

Chapter 25

Esophageal Cancer

The Esophagus

The esophagus is in the chest. It's about 10 inches long. This organ is part of the digestive tract. Food moves from the mouth through the esophagus to the stomach. The esophagus is a muscular tube. The wall of the esophagus has several layers:

- **Inner Layer Or Lining (Mucosa):** The lining of the esophagus is moist so that food can pass to the stomach.

- **Submucosa:** The glands in this layer make mucus. Mucus keeps the esophagus moist.

- **Muscle Layer:** The muscles push the food down to the stomach.

- **Outer Layer:** The outer layer covers the esophagus.

Growths in the wall of the esophagus can be benign (not cancer) or malignant (cancer). The smooth inner wall may have an abnormal rough area, an area of tiny bumps, or a tumor. Benign growths are not as harmful as malignant growths.

Esophageal cancer begins in cells in the inner layer of the esophagus. Over time, the cancer may invade more deeply into the esophagus and nearby tissues.

About This Chapter: Text in this chapter is excerpted from "What You Need to Know about Cancer of the Esophagus," National Cancer Institute, November 21, 2008.

Types Of Esophageal Cancer

There are two main types of esophageal cancer. Both types are diagnosed, treated, and managed in similar ways. The two most common types are named for how the cancer cells look under a microscope. Both types begin in cells in the inner lining of the esophagus:

- **Adenocarcinoma Of The Esophagus:** This type is usually found in the lower part of the esophagus, near the stomach. In the United States, adenocarcinoma is the most common type of esophageal cancer. It's been increasing since the 1970s.

- **Squamous Cell Carcinoma Of The Esophagus:** This type is usually found in the upper part of the esophagus. This type is becoming less common among Americans. Around the world, however, squamous cell carcinoma is the most common type.

Risk Factors

Doctors can seldom explain why one person develops esophageal cancer and another doesn't. However, we do know that people with certain risk factors are more likely than others to develop esophageal cancer. A risk factor is something that may increase the chance of getting a disease.

Studies have found the following risk factors for esophageal cancer:

- **Age:** Age is the main risk factor for esophageal cancer. The chance of getting this disease goes up as you get older. In the United States, most people are 65 years of age or older when they are diagnosed with esophageal cancer.

✤ It's A Fact!!

Smoking is a risk factor for esophageal cancer. When compared with people who do not smoke, people who do smoke are more likely to develop esophageal cancer. In addition, drinkers who have more than three alcoholic drinks each day and who smoke are at a much higher risk than similar drinkers who don't smoke.

- **Gender:** In the United States, men are more than three times as likely as women to develop esophageal cancer.

- **Smoking:** People who smoke are more likely than people who don't smoke to develop esophageal cancer.

- **Heavy Drinking:** People who have more than three alcoholic drinks each day are more likely than people who don't drink to develop squamous cell carcinoma of the esophagus. Heavy drinkers who smoke are at a much higher risk than heavy drinkers who don't smoke. In other words, these two factors act together to increase the risk even more.

- **Diet:** Studies suggest that having a diet that is low in fruits and vegetables may increase the risk of esophageal cancer. However, results from diet studies don't always agree, and more research is needed to better understand how diet affects the risk of developing esophageal cancer.

- **Obesity:** Being obese increases the risk of adenocarcinoma of the esophagus.

- **Acid Reflux:** Acid reflux is the abnormal backward flow of stomach acid into the esophagus. Reflux is very common. A symptom of reflux is heartburn, but some people don't have symptoms. The stomach acid can damage the tissue of the esophagus. After many years of reflux, this tissue damage may lead to adenocarcinoma of the esophagus in some people.

- **Barrett Esophagus:** Acid reflux may damage the esophagus and over time cause a condition known as Barrett esophagus. The cells in the lower part of the esophagus are abnormal. Most people who have Barrett esophagus don't know it. The presence of Barrett esophagus increases the risk of adenocarcinoma of the esophagus. It's a greater risk factor than acid reflux alone.

Many other possible risk factors (such as smokeless tobacco) have been studied. Researchers continue to study these possible risk factors.

Having a risk factor doesn't mean that a person will develop cancer of the esophagus. Most people who have risk factors never develop esophageal cancer.

Symptoms

Early esophageal cancer may not cause symptoms. As the cancer grows, the most common symptoms are the following:

- Food gets stuck in the esophagus, and food may come back up
- Pain when swallowing
- Pain in the chest or back
- Weight loss
- Heartburn
- A hoarse voice or cough that doesn't go away within two weeks

These symptoms may be caused by esophageal cancer or other health problems. If you have any of these symptoms, you should tell your doctor so that problems can be diagnosed and treated as early as possible.

Diagnosis

If you have a symptom that suggests esophageal cancer, your doctor must find out whether it's really due to cancer or to some other cause. The doctor gives you a physical exam and asks about your personal and family health history. You may have blood tests. Some additional tests you also may have include the following:

- **Barium Swallow:** After you drink a barium solution, you have x-rays taken of your esophagus and stomach.
- **Endoscopy:** The doctor uses a thin, lighted tube (endoscope) to look down your esophagus.
- **Biopsy:** Usually, cancer begins in the inner layer of the esophagus. The doctor uses an endoscope to remove tissue from the esophagus. A pathologist checks the tissue under a microscope for cancer cells. A biopsy is the only sure way to know if cancer cells are present.

Staging

If the biopsy shows that you have cancer, your doctor needs to learn the extent (stage) of the disease to help you choose the best treatment. Staging is a careful attempt to find out how deeply the cancer invades the walls of the esophagus, whether the cancer invades nearby tissues, whether the cancer has spread, and if so, to what parts of the body.

When esophageal cancer spreads, it's often found in nearby lymph nodes. If cancer has reached these nodes, it may also have spread to other lymph nodes, the bones, or other organs. Also, esophageal cancer may spread to the liver and lungs.

When cancer spreads from its original place to another part of the body, the new tumor has the same kind of abnormal cells and the same name as the primary tumor. For example, if esophageal cancer spreads to the liver, the cancer cells in the liver are actually esophageal cancer cells. The disease is metastatic esophageal cancer, not liver cancer. For that reason, it's treated as esophageal cancer, not liver cancer. Doctors call the new tumor "distant" or metastatic disease.

Treatment

People with esophageal cancer have several treatment options. The options are surgery, radiation therapy, chemotherapy, or a combination of these treatments. For example, radiation therapy and chemotherapy may be given before or after surgery.

Surgery

There are several types of surgery for esophageal cancer. The type depends mainly on where the cancer is located. The surgeon may remove the whole esophagus or only the part that has the cancer. Usually, the surgeon removes the section of the esophagus with the cancer, lymph nodes, and nearby soft tissues. Part or all of the stomach may also be removed.

The surgeon makes incisions into your chest and abdomen to remove the cancer. In most cases, the surgeon pulls up the stomach and joins it to the remaining part of the esophagus. Or a piece of intestine may be used to connect the stomach to the remaining part of the esophagus. The surgeon may use either a piece of small intestine or large intestine. If the stomach was removed, a piece of intestine is used to join the remaining part of the esophagus to the small intestine.

During surgery, the surgeon may place a feeding tube into your small intestine. This tube helps you get enough nutrition while you heal.

You may have pain for the first few days after surgery. However, medicine will help control the pain. Before surgery, you should discuss the plan for pain relief with your health care team. After surgery, your team can adjust the plan if you need more relief.

Your health care team will watch for signs of food leaking from the newly joined parts of your digestive tract. They will also watch for pneumonia or other infections, breathing problems, bleeding, or other problems that may require treatment.

The time it takes to heal after surgery is different for everyone and depends on the type of surgery. You may be in the hospital for at least one week.

Radiation Therapy

Radiation therapy (also called radiotherapy) uses high-energy rays to kill cancer cells. It affects cells only in the treated area.

Radiation therapy may be used before or after surgery. Or it may be used instead of surgery. Radiation therapy is usually given with chemotherapy to treat esophageal cancer.

Doctors use two types of radiation therapy to treat esophageal cancer: external radiation therapy and internal radiation therapy. Some people receive both types.

- **External Radiation Therapy:** The radiation comes from a large machine outside the body. The machine aims radiation at your cancer. You may go to a hospital or clinic for treatment. Treatments are usually five days a week for several weeks.

- **Internal Radiation Therapy (Brachytherapy):** The doctor numbs your throat with an anesthetic spray and gives you medicine to help you relax. The doctor puts a tube into your esophagus. The radiation comes from the tube. Once the tube is removed, no radioactivity is left in your body. Usually, only a single treatment is done.

Side effects depend mainly on the dose and type of radiation. External radiation therapy to the chest and abdomen may cause a sore throat, pain similar to heartburn, or pain in the stomach or the intestine. You may have nausea and diarrhea. Your health care team can give you medicines to prevent or control these problems.

Also, your skin in the treated area may become red, dry, and tender. You may lose hair in the treated area. A much less common side effect of radiation therapy aimed at the chest is harm to the lung, heart, or spinal cord.

You are likely to be very tired during radiation therapy, especially in the later weeks of external radiation therapy. You may also continue to feel very tired for a few weeks after radiation therapy is completed. Resting is important, but doctors usually advise patients to try to stay as active as they can.

Radiation therapy can lead to problems with swallowing. For example, sometimes radiation therapy can harm the esophagus and make it painful for you to swallow. Or, the radiation may cause the esophagus to narrow. Before radiation therapy, a plastic tube may be inserted into the esophagus to keep it open. If radiation therapy leads to a problem with swallowing, it may be hard to eat well.

♣ It's A Fact!!
Supportive Care

Esophageal cancer and its treatment can lead to other health problems. You can have supportive care before, during, or after cancer treatment.

Supportive care is treatment to control pain and other symptoms, to relieve the side effects of therapy, and to help you cope with the feelings that a diagnosis of cancer can bring. You may receive supportive care to prevent or control these problems and to improve your comfort and quality of life during treatment.

It's normal to feel sad, anxious, or confused after a diagnosis of a serious illness. Some people find it helpful to talk about their feelings.

Chemotherapy

Most people with esophageal cancer get chemotherapy. Chemotherapy uses drugs to destroy cancer cells. The drugs for esophageal cancer are usually given through a vein (intravenous). You may have your treatment in a clinic, at the doctor's office, or at home. Some people need to stay in the hospital for treatment.

Chemotherapy is usually given in cycles. Each cycle has a treatment period followed by a rest period.

The side effects depend mainly on which drugs are given and how much. Chemotherapy kills fast-growing cancer cells, but the drug can also harm normal cells that divide rapidly.

Nutrition

It's important to meet your nutrition needs before, during, and after cancer treatment. You need the right amount of calories, protein, vitamins, and minerals. Getting the right nutrition can help you feel better and have more energy.

However, when you have esophageal cancer, it may be hard to eat for many reasons. You may be uncomfortable or tired, and you may not feel like eating. Also, the cancer may make it hard to swallow food. If you're getting chemotherapy, you may find that foods don't taste as good as they used to. You also may have side effects of treatment such as poor appetite, nausea, vomiting, or diarrhea.

If you develop problems with eating, there are a number of ways to meet your nutrition needs. A registered dietitian can help you figure out a way to get enough calories, protein, vitamins, and minerals.

Follow-Up Care

You'll need checkups after treatment for esophageal cancer. Checkups help ensure that any changes in your health are noted and treated if needed. Checkups may include a physical exam, blood tests, chest x-ray, CT scans, endoscopy, or other tests.

Chapter 26

Kidney Cancer

The Kidneys

The kidneys are a pair of organs on either side of the spine in the lower abdomen. Each kidney is about the size of a fist. The kidneys are part of the urinary tract. They make urine by removing wastes and extra water from the blood. They also make substances that help control blood pressure and the production of red blood cells.

Several types of cancer can start in the kidney. This chapter is about renal cell cancer, the most common type of kidney cancer in adults. This type is sometimes called renal adenocarcinoma or hypernephroma. Another type of cancer, transitional cell carcinoma, affects the renal pelvis. It is similar to bladder cancer and is often treated like bladder cancer. Wilms tumor is the most common type of childhood kidney cancer. It is different from adult kidney cancer and requires different treatment.

When kidney cancer spreads outside the kidney, cancer cells are often found in nearby lymph nodes. Kidney cancer also may spread to the lungs, bones, or liver. And it may spread from one kidney to the other.

About This Chapter: Text in this chapter is excerpted from "What You Need to Know about Kidney Cancer," National Cancer Institute, March 30, 2004.

Who's At Risk For Kidney Cancer?

Kidney cancer develops most often in people over 40, but no one knows the exact causes of this disease. Doctors can seldom explain why one person develops kidney cancer and another does not. However, it is clear that kidney cancer is not contagious. No one can "catch" the disease from another person.

Research has shown that people with certain risk factors are more likely than others to develop kidney cancer. A risk factor is anything that increases a person's chance of developing a disease.

Studies have found the following risk factors for kidney cancer:

- **Smoking:** Cigarette smoking is a major risk factor. Cigarette smokers are twice as likely as nonsmokers to develop kidney cancer. Cigar smoking also may increase the risk of this disease.

- **Obesity:** People who are obese have an increased risk of kidney cancer.

- **High Blood Pressure:** High blood pressure increases the risk of kidney cancer.

- **Long-Term Dialysis:** Dialysis is a treatment for people whose kidneys do not work well. It removes wastes from the blood. Being on dialysis for many years is a risk factor for kidney cancer.

- **Von Hippel-Lindau (VHL) Syndrome:** VHL is a rare disease that runs in some families. It is caused by changes in the VHL gene. An abnormal VHL gene increases the risk of kidney cancer.

- **Occupation:** Some people have a higher risk of getting kidney cancer because they come in contact with certain chemicals or substances in their workplace. Coke oven workers in the iron and steel industry are at risk. Workers exposed to asbestos or cadmium also may be at risk.

♣ It's A Fact!!

Compared with nonsmokers, cigarette smokers are twice as likely to develop kidney cancer. Cigar smoking also may increase the risk.

- **Gender:** Males are more likely than females to be diagnosed with kidney cancer. Each year in the United States, about 20,000 men and 12,000 women learn they have kidney cancer.

Most people who have these risk factors do not get kidney cancer. On the other hand, most people who do get the disease have no known risk factors. People who think they may be at risk should discuss this concern with their doctor. The doctor may be able to suggest ways to reduce the risk and can plan an appropriate schedule for checkups.

Symptoms

Common symptoms of kidney cancer include the following:

- Blood in the urine (making the urine slightly rusty to deep red)
- Pain in the side that does not go away
- A lump or mass in the side or the abdomen
- Weight loss
- Fever
- Feeling very tired or having a general feeling of poor health

Most often, these symptoms do not mean cancer. An infection, a cyst, or another problem also can cause the same symptoms. A person with any of these symptoms should see a doctor so that any problem can be diagnosed and treated as early as possible.

Diagnosis

If a patient has symptoms that suggest kidney cancer, the doctor may perform one or more of the following procedures:

- **Physical Exam:** The doctor checks general signs of health and tests for fever and high blood pressure. The doctor also feels the abdomen and side for tumors.
- **Urine Tests:** Urine is checked for blood and other signs of disease.
- **Blood Tests:** The lab checks the blood to see how well the kidneys are working. The lab may check the level of several substances, such

as creatinine. A high level of creatinine may mean the kidneys are not doing their job.

- **Intravenous Pyelogram (IVP):** The doctor injects dye into a vein in the arm. The dye travels through the body and collects in the kidneys. The dye makes them show up on x-rays. A series of x-rays then tracks the dye as it moves through the kidneys to the ureters and bladder. The x-rays can show a kidney tumor or other problems.

- **CT Scan (CAT Scan):** An x-ray machine linked to a computer takes a series of detailed pictures of the kidneys. The patient may receive an injection of dye so the kidneys show up clearly in the pictures. A CT scan can show a kidney tumor.

- **Ultrasound Test:** The ultrasound device uses sound waves that people cannot hear. The waves bounce off the kidneys, and a computer uses the echoes to create a picture called a sonogram. A solid tumor or cyst shows up on a sonogram.

- **Biopsy:** In some cases, the doctor may do a biopsy. A biopsy is the removal of tissue to look for cancer cells. The doctor inserts a thin needle through the skin into the kidney to remove a small amount of tissue. The doctor may use ultrasound or x-rays to guide the needle. A pathologist uses a microscope to look for cancer cells in the tissue.

- **Surgery:** In most cases, based on the results of the CT scan, ultrasound, and x-rays, the doctor has enough information to recommend surgery to remove part or all of the kidney. A pathologist makes the final diagnosis by examining the tissue under a microscope.

To plan the best treatment, the doctor also needs to know the stage (extent) of the disease. The stage is based on the size of the tumor, whether the cancer has spread and, if so, to what parts of the body.

Treatment

The doctor may refer the patient to a specialist, or the patient may ask for a referral. Specialists who treat kidney cancer include doctors who specialize in diseases of the urinary system (urologists) and doctors who specialize in cancer (medical oncologists and radiation oncologists). Treatment depends mainly on the stage of disease and the patient's general health and age.

People with kidney cancer may have surgery, arterial embolization, radiation therapy, biological therapy, or chemotherapy. Some may have a combination of treatments.

At any stage of disease, people with kidney cancer may have treatment to control pain and other symptoms, to relieve the side effects of therapy, and to ease emotional and practical problems. This kind of treatment is called supportive care, symptom management, or palliative care.

A patient may want to talk to the doctor about taking part in a clinical trial, a research study of new treatment methods.

Surgery

Surgery is the most common treatment for kidney cancer. It is a type of local therapy. It treats cancer in the kidney and the area close to the tumor.

An operation to remove the kidney is called a nephrectomy. There are several types of nephrectomies. The type depends mainly on the stage of the tumor. The doctor can explain each operation and discuss which is most suitable for the patient.

- **Radical Nephrectomy:** Kidney cancer is usually treated with radical nephrectomy. The surgeon removes the entire kidney along with the adrenal gland and some tissue around the kidney. Some lymph nodes in the area also may be removed.

♣ It's A Fact!!

Because treatment for kidney cancer may damage healthy cells and tissues, unwanted side effects are common. These side effects depend mainly on the type and extent of the treatment. Side effects may not be the same for each person, and they may change from one treatment session to the next. Before treatment starts, the health care team will explain possible side effects and suggest ways to help the patient manage them.

- **Simple Nephrectomy:** The surgeon removes only the kidney. Some people with stage I kidney cancer may have a simple nephrectomy.

- **Partial Nephrectomy:** The surgeon removes only the part of the kidney that contains the tumor. This type of surgery may be used when the person has only one kidney, or when the cancer affects both kidneys. Also, a person with a small kidney tumor (less than four centimeters) may have this type of surgery.

Arterial Embolization

Arterial embolization is a type of local therapy that shrinks the tumor. Sometimes it is done before an operation to make surgery easier. When surgery is not possible, embolization may be used to help relieve the symptoms of kidney cancer. The doctor inserts a narrow tube (catheter) into a blood vessel in the leg. The tube is passed up to the main blood vessel (renal artery) that supplies blood to the kidney. The doctor injects a substance into the blood vessel to block the flow of blood into the kidney. The blockage prevents the tumor from getting oxygen and other substances it needs to grow.

Radiation Therapy

Radiation therapy (also called radiotherapy) is another type of local therapy. It uses high-energy rays to kill cancer cells. It affects cancer cells only in the treated area. A large machine directs radiation at the body. The patient has treatment at the hospital or clinic, five days a week for several weeks.

A small number of patients have radiation therapy before surgery to shrink the tumor. Some have it after surgery to kill cancer cells that may remain in the area. People who cannot have surgery may have radiation therapy to relieve pain and other problems caused by the cancer.

Biological Therapy

Biological therapy is a type of systemic therapy. It uses substances that travel through the bloodstream, reaching and affecting cells all over the body. Biological therapy uses the body's natural ability (immune system) to fight cancer.

Chemotherapy

Chemotherapy is also a type of systemic therapy. Anticancer drugs enter the bloodstream and travel throughout the body. Although useful for many other cancers, anticancer drugs have shown limited use against kidney cancer. However, many doctors are studying new drugs and new combinations that may prove more helpful.

Follow-Up Care

Follow-up care after treatment for kidney cancer is important. Even when the cancer seems to have been completely removed or destroyed, the disease sometimes returns because cancer cells can remain in the body after treatment. The doctor monitors the recovery of the person treated for kidney cancer and checks for recurrence of cancer. Checkups help ensure that any changes in health are noted. The patient may have lab tests, chest x-rays, CT scans, or other tests.

Chapter 27

Laryngeal Cancer

The Larynx

The larynx is an organ at the front of your neck. It is also called the voice box. It is about two inches long and two inches wide. It is above the windpipe (trachea). Below and behind the larynx is the esophagus.

The larynx has two bands of muscle that form the vocal cords. The cartilage at the front of the larynx is sometimes called the Adam's apple. The larynx has three main parts:

- The top part of the larynx is the supraglottis.

- The glottis is in the middle. Your vocal cords are in the glottis.

- The subglottis is at the bottom. The subglottis connects to the windpipe.

The larynx plays a role in breathing, swallowing, and talking. The larynx acts like a valve over the windpipe. The valve opens and closes to allow breathing, swallowing, and speaking. When you breathe, the vocal cords relax and open. When you hold your breath, the vocal cords shut tightly. The larynx protects the windpipe. When you swallow, a flap called the epiglottis covers the opening of your larynx to keep food out of your lungs. The food passes through

About This Chapter: Text in this chapter is excerpted from "What You Need to Know about Cancer of the Larynx," National Cancer Institute, May 5, 2003.

the esophagus on its way from your mouth to your stomach. The larynx also produces the sound of your voice. When you talk, your vocal cords tighten and move closer together. Air from your lungs is forced between them and makes them vibrate. This makes the sound of your voice. Your tongue, lips, and teeth form this sound into words.

Cancer of the larynx also may be called laryngeal cancer. It can develop in any part of the larynx. Most cancers of the larynx begin in the glottis. The inner walls of the larynx are lined with cells called squamous cells. Almost all laryngeal cancers begin in these cells. These cancers are called squamous cell carcinomas.

If cancer of the larynx spreads (metastasizes), the cancer cells often spread to nearby lymph nodes in the neck. The cancer cells can also spread to the back of the tongue, other parts of the throat and neck, the lungs, and other parts of the body. When this happens, the new tumor has the same kind of abnormal cells as the primary tumor in the larynx. For example, if cancer of the larynx spreads to the lungs, the cancer cells in the lungs are actually laryngeal cancer cells. The disease is called metastatic cancer of the larynx, not lung cancer. It is treated as cancer of the larynx, not lung cancer. Doctors sometimes call the new tumor "distant" disease.

Cancer Of The Larynx: Who's At Risk?

No one knows the exact causes of cancer of the larynx. Doctors cannot explain why one person gets this disease and another does not. We do know that cancer is not contagious. You cannot "catch" cancer from another person.

People with certain risk factors are more likely to get cancer of the larynx. A risk factor is anything that increases your chance of developing this disease.

Studies have found the following risk factors:

Age: Cancer of the larynx occurs most often in people over the age of 55.

Gender: Men are four times more likely than women to get cancer of the larynx.

Race: African Americans are more likely than whites to be diagnosed with cancer of the larynx.

Smoking: Smokers are far more likely than nonsmokers to get cancer of the larynx. The risk is even higher for smokers who drink alcohol heavily.

Alcohol: People who drink alcohol are more likely to develop laryngeal cancer than people who don't drink. The risk increases with the amount of alcohol that is consumed. The risk also increases if the person drinks alcohol and also smokes tobacco.

Head And Neck Cancer: Almost one in four people who have had head and neck cancer will develop a second primary head and neck cancer.

Occupation: Workers exposed to sulfuric acid mist or nickel have an increased risk of laryngeal cancer. Also, working with asbestos can increase the risk of this disease. Asbestos workers should follow work and safety rules to avoid inhaling asbestos fibers.

Other studies suggest that having certain viruses or a diet low in vitamin A may increase the chance of getting cancer of the larynx. Another risk factor is having gastroesophageal reflux disease (GERD), which causes stomach acid to flow up into the esophagus.

Most people who have these risk factors do not get cancer of the larynx. If you are concerned about your chance of getting cancer of the larynx, you should discuss this concern with your health care provider. Your health care provider may suggest ways to reduce your risk and can plan an appropriate schedule for checkups.

❖ **It's A Fact!!**
People who stop smoking can greatly decrease their risk of cancer of the larynx, as well as cancer of the lung, mouth, pancreas, bladder, and esophagus. Also, quitting smoking reduces the chance that someone with cancer of the larynx will get a second cancer in the head and neck region. (Cancer of the larynx is part of a group of cancers called head and neck cancers.)

Symptoms

The symptoms of cancer of the larynx depend mainly on the size of the tumor and where it is in the larynx. Symptoms may include the following:

- Hoarseness or other voice changes
- A lump in the neck
- A sore throat or feeling that something is stuck in your throat
- A cough that does not go away
- Problems breathing
- Bad breath
- An earache
- Weight loss

These symptoms may be caused by cancer or by other, less serious problems. Only a doctor can tell for sure.

Diagnosis

If you have symptoms of cancer of the larynx, the doctor may do some or all of the following exams:

- **Physical Exam:** The doctor will feel your neck and check your thyroid, larynx, and lymph nodes for abnormal lumps or swelling. To see your throat, the doctor may press down on your tongue.

- **Indirect Laryngoscopy:** The doctor looks down your throat using a small, long-handled mirror to check for abnormal areas and to see if your vocal cords move as they should. This test does not hurt. The doctor may spray a local anesthesia in your throat to keep you from gagging. This exam is done in the doctor's office.

- **Direct Laryngoscopy:** The doctor inserts a thin, lighted tube called a laryngoscope through your nose or mouth. As the tube goes down your throat, the doctor can look at areas that cannot be seen with a mirror. A local anesthetic eases discomfort and prevents gagging. You may also receive a mild sedative to help you relax. Sometimes the doctor uses general anesthesia to put a person to sleep. This exam may be done in a doctor's office, an outpatient clinic, or a hospital.

- **CT Scan:** An x-ray machine linked to a computer takes a series of detailed pictures of the neck area. You may receive an injection of a special dye so your larynx shows up clearly in the pictures. From the CT scan, the doctor may see tumors in your larynx or elsewhere in your neck.

- **Biopsy:** If an exam shows an abnormal area, the doctor may remove a small sample of tissue. Removing tissue to look for cancer cells is called a biopsy. For a biopsy, you receive local or general anesthesia, and the doctor removes tissue samples through a laryngoscope. A pathologist then looks at the tissue under a microscope to check for cancer cells. A biopsy is the only sure way to know if a tumor is cancerous.

Treatment

Your doctor may refer you to a specialist who treats cancer of the larynx, such as a surgeon, otolaryngologist (an ear, nose, and throat doctor), radiation oncologist, or medical oncologist. You can also ask your doctor for a referral. Treatment usually begins within a few weeks of the diagnosis. Usually, there is time to talk to your doctor about treatment choices, get a second opinion, and learn more about the disease before making a treatment decision.

The doctor can describe your treatment choices and the results you can expect for each treatment option. You will want to consider how treatment may change the way you look, breathe, and talk. You and your doctor can work together to develop a treatment plan that meets your needs and personal values.

The choice of treatment depends on a number of factors, including your general health, where in the larynx the cancer began, the size of the tumor, and whether the cancer has spread.

You may want to talk with the doctor about taking part in a clinical trial, a research study of new treatment methods. Clinical trials are an important option. Patients who join trials have the first chance to benefit from new treatments that have shown promise in earlier research.

Cancer of the larynx may be treated with radiation therapy, surgery, or chemotherapy. Some patients have a combination of therapies. Radiation therapy (also called radiotherapy) uses high-energy x-rays to kill cancer cells. Laryngeal cancer may be treated with radiation therapy alone or in combination with surgery or chemotherapy.

Radiation Therapy

The rays are aimed at the tumor and the tissue around it. Radiation therapy is local therapy. It affects cells only in the treated area. Treatments are usually given five days a week for five to eight weeks. Radiation therapy is used alone for small tumors or for patients who cannot have surgery. Radiation therapy may be used to shrink a large tumor before surgery or to destroy cancer cells that may remain in the area after surgery. If a tumor grows back after surgery, it is often treated with radiation. Radiation therapy may also be used before, during, or after chemotherapy.

After radiation therapy, some people need feeding tubes placed into the abdomen. The feeding tube is usually temporary.

Surgery

Surgery is an operation in which a doctor removes the cancer using a scalpel or laser while the patient is asleep. When patients need surgery, the type of operation depends mainly on the size and exact location of the tumor. There are several types of laryngectomy (surgery to remove part or all of the larynx):

- **Total laryngectomy:** The surgeon removes the entire larynx.

> **✔ Quick Tip**
>
> If you smoke, a good way to prepare for treatment is to stop smoking. Studies show that treatment is more likely to be successful for people who don't smoke. Your doctor may be able to suggest ways to help you stop smoking.

- **Partial laryngectomy (hemilaryngectomy):** The surgeon removes part of the larynx.

- **Supraglottic laryngectomy:** The surgeon takes out the supraglottis, the top part of the larynx.

- **Cordectomy:** The surgeon removes one or both vocal cords.

Sometimes the surgeon also removes the lymph nodes in the neck. This is called lymph node dissection. The surgeon also may remove the thyroid.

During surgery for cancer of the larynx, the surgeon may need to make a stoma. (This surgery is called a tracheostomy.) The stoma is a new airway through an opening in the front of the neck. Air enters and leaves the windpipe (trachea) and lungs through this opening. A tracheostomy tube, also called a trach ("trake") tube, keeps the new airway open. For many patients, the stoma is temporary. It is needed only until the patient recovers from surgery.

After surgery, some people may need a temporary feeding tube.

Chemotherapy

Chemotherapy is the use of drugs to kill cancer cells. Your doctor may suggest one drug or a combination of drugs. The drugs for cancer of the larynx are usually given by injection into the bloodstream. The drugs enter the bloodstream and travel throughout the body.

Side Effects Of Cancer Treatment

Treatments that remove or destroy cancer cells are likely to damage healthy cells, too. That's why treatments often cause side effects. Side effects may not be the same for each person, and they may even change from one treatment session to the next. Before treatment starts, your health care team will explain possible side effects and how they can be managed. It may help to know that although some side effects may not go away completely, most of them become less troubling.

Radiation Therapy

People treated with radiation therapy may have some or all of these side effects:

- Dry mouth

- Sore throat or mouth

- Delayed healing after dental care

- Tooth decay

- Changes in sense of taste and smell

- Fatigue

- Changes in voice quality

- Skin changes in treated area

Surgery

> ♣ **It's A Fact!!**
>
> **Living With A Stoma**
>
> Learning to live with the changes brought about by cancer of the larynx is a special challenge. The medical team will make every effort to help you return to your normal routine as soon as possible. If you have a stoma, you will need to learn how to care for it.

People who have surgery may have any of these side effects:

- Pain

- Low energy

- Swelling in the throat

- Increased mucus production

- Numbness, stiffness, or weakness

- Changes in physical appearance

- Tracheostomy

Chemotherapy

The side effects of chemotherapy depend mainly on the specific drugs and the dose. In general, anticancer drugs affect cells that divide rapidly, including blood cells, cells in hair roots, and cells that line the digestive tract.

Nutrition

Some people who have had treatment for cancer of the larynx may lose their interest in food. Soreness and changes in smell and taste may make eating difficult. Yet good nutrition is important. Eating well means getting enough calories and protein to prevent weight loss, regain strength, and rebuild healthy tissues.

If eating is difficult because your mouth is dry from radiation therapy, you may want to try soft, bland foods moistened with sauces or gravies. Thick soups, puddings, and milkshakes often are easier to swallow. The nurse and the dietitian will help you choose the right foods.

After surgery or radiation therapy, some people need feeding tubes placed into the abdomen. Most people slowly return to a regular diet. Learning to swallow again may take some practice with the help of a nurse or speech pathologist. Some people find liquids easier to swallow; others do better with solid foods. You will find what works best for you.

Learning To Speak Again

Talking is part of nearly everything we do, so it's natural to be scared if your voice box must be removed. Losing the ability to talk—even for a short time—is hard. Patients and their families and friends need understanding and support during this time.

Within a week or so after a partial laryngectomy, you will be able to talk in the usual way. After a total laryngectomy, however, you must learn to speak in a new way. A speech pathologist usually meets with you before surgery to explain the methods that can be used. In many cases, speech lessons start before you leave the hospital.

Until you begin to talk again, it is important to have other ways to communicate. Here are some ideas that you may find helpful:

- Keep pads of paper and pens or pencils in your pocket or purse.

- Use a typewriter, computer, or other electronic device. Your words can be printed on paper, displayed on a screen, or produced in a male or female voice.

- Carry a small dictionary or a picture book and point to the words you need.

- Write notes on a "magic slate" (a toy with a plastic sheet that covers black wax; lifting the plastic erases the sheet).

The health care team can help patients learn new ways to speak. It takes practice and patience to learn techniques such as esophageal speech or tracheoesophageal puncture speech, and not everyone is successful. How quickly a person learns, how understandable the speech is, and how natural the new voice sounds depend on the extent of the surgery on the larynx.

✎ What's It Mean?

Esophageal Speech: A way of speaking in which you force air into the top of your esophagus and then push it out again. The puff of air is like a burp. It vibrates the walls of the throat, making sound for the new voice. The tongue, lips, and teeth form words as the sound passes through the mouth. This type of speech sounds low pitched and gruff, but it usually sounds more like a natural voice than speech made by a mechanical larynx. There is also no device to carry around, so your hands are free.

Tracheoesophageal Puncture (TEP): A way of speaking in which the surgeon makes an opening between the trachea and the esophagus. The opening is made at the time of initial surgery or later. A small plastic or silicone valve fits into this opening. The valve keeps food out of the trachea. After TEP, patients can cover their stoma with a finger and force air into the esophagus through the valve. The air produces sound by making the walls of the throat vibrate. The sound is a lot like natural speech.

Mechanical Speech: A way of speaking in which a device, which may be powered by batteries (electrolarynx) or by air (pneumatic larynx), is used. One kind of electrolarynx looks like a small flashlight. It makes a humming sound. You hold the device against your neck, and the sound travels through your neck to your mouth. Another type of electrolarynx has a flexible plastic tube that carries sound into your mouth from a hand-held device. There are also devices that are built into a denture or retainer and can be worn inside your mouth and operated by a hand-held remote control. A pneumatic larynx is held over the stoma and uses air from the lungs instead of batteries to make it vibrate. The sound it makes travels to the mouth through a plastic tube.

Follow-Up Care

Follow-up care is important after treatment for cancer of the larynx. Regular checkups ensure that any changes in health are noted. Problems can be found and treated as soon as possible. The doctor will check closely to be sure that the cancer has not returned. Checkups include exams of the stoma, neck, and throat. From time to time, the doctor may do a complete physical exam and take x-rays. If you had radiation therapy or a partial laryngectomy, the doctor will also examine you with a laryngoscope.

Treatments for laryngeal cancer can affect the thyroid. A blood test can tell if the thyroid is making enough thyroid hormone. If the level is low, you may need to take thyroid hormone pills.

People who have laryngeal cancer have a chance of developing a new cancer in the mouth, throat, or other areas of the head and neck. This is especially true for those who are smokers or drink alcohol heavily.

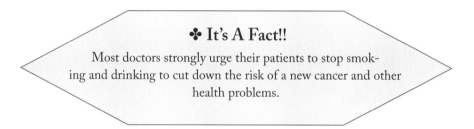

❖ It's A Fact!!
Most doctors strongly urge their patients to stop smoking and drinking to cut down the risk of a new cancer and other health problems.

Chapter 28

Leukemia

What Is Leukemia?

Leukemia is cancer that starts in the tissue that forms blood. To understand cancer, it helps to know how normal blood cells form.

Normal Blood Cells

Most blood cells develop from cells in the bone marrow called stem cells. Bone marrow is the soft material in the center of most bones. Stem cells mature into different kinds of blood cells. Each kind has a special job:

- White blood cells help fight infection. There are several types of white blood cells.

- Red blood cells carry oxygen to tissues throughout the body.

- Platelets help form blood clots that control bleeding.

White blood cells, red blood cells, and platelets are made from stem cells as the body needs them. When cells grow old or get damaged, they die, and new cells take their place.

About This Chapter: Text in this chapter is excerpted from "What You Need to Know about Leukemia," National Cancer Institute, November 25, 2008.

Stem cells mature into different types of white blood cells. First, a stem cell matures into either a myeloid stem cell or a lymphoid stem cell. A myeloid stem cell matures into a myeloid blast. The blast can form a red blood cell, platelets, or one of several types of white blood cells. A lymphoid stem cell matures into a lymphoid blast. The blast can form one of several types of white blood cells, such as B cells or T cells.

The white blood cells that form from myeloid blasts are different from the white blood cells that form from lymphoid blasts.

Most blood cells mature in the bone marrow and then move into the blood vessels. Blood flowing through the blood vessels and heart is called the peripheral blood.

Leukemia Cells

In a person with leukemia, the bone marrow makes abnormal white blood cells. The abnormal cells are leukemia cells. Unlike normal blood cells, leukemia cells don't die when they should. They may crowd out normal white blood cells, red blood cells, and platelets. This makes it hard for normal blood cells to do their work.

Types Of Leukemia

The types of leukemia can be grouped based on how quickly the disease develops and gets worse. Leukemia is either chronic (which usually gets worse slowly) or acute (which usually gets worse quickly).

There are four common types of leukemia:

- Chronic lymphocytic leukemia
- Chronic myeloid leukemia
- Acute lymphocytic (lymphoblastic) leukemia
- Acute myeloid leukemia

Risk Factors

No one knows the exact causes of leukemia. However, research shows that certain risk factors increase the chance that a person will get this disease. The risk factors may be different for the different types of leukemia:

- **Radiation:** People exposed to very high levels of radiation are much more likely than others to get acute myeloid leukemia, chronic myeloid leukemia, or acute lymphocytic leukemia.

- **Smoking:** Smoking cigarettes increases the risk of acute myeloid leukemia.

- **Benzene:** Exposure to benzene in the workplace can cause acute myeloid leukemia. It may also cause chronic myeloid leukemia or acute lymphocytic leukemia. Benzene is used widely in the chemical industry. It's also found in cigarette smoke and gasoline.

- **Chemotherapy:** Cancer patients treated with certain types of cancer-fighting drugs sometimes later get acute myeloid leukemia or acute lymphocytic leukemia.

- **Down Syndrome:** Down syndrome and certain other inherited diseases increase the risk of developing acute leukemia.

- **Myelodysplastic Syndrome**: People with myelodysplastic syndrome and certain blood disorders are at increased risk of acute myeloid leukemia.

- **Human T-Cell Leukemia Virus Type I (HTLV-I):** People with HTLV-I infection are at increased risk of a rare type of leukemia known as adult T-cell leukemia. Although the HTLV-I virus may cause this rare disease, adult T-cell leukemia and other types of leukemia are not contagious.

- **Family History:** It's rare for more than one person in a family to have leukemia. When it does happen, it's most likely to involve chronic lymphocytic leukemia. However, only a few people with chronic lymphocytic leukemia have a father, mother, brother, sister, or child who also has the disease.

Having one or more risk factors does not mean that a person will get leukemia. Most people who have risk factors never develop the disease.

Symptoms

Like all blood cells, leukemia cells travel through the body. The symptoms of leukemia depend on the number of leukemia cells and where these cells collect in the body. People with chronic leukemia may not have symptoms. The doctor may find the disease during a routine blood test.

❖ It's A Fact!!

Smoking cigarettes increases the risk of acute myeloid leukemia. In addition, cigarette smoke contains benzene, which is a risk factor for chronic myeloid leukemia and acute lymphocytic leukemia.

People with acute leukemia usually go to their doctor because they feel sick. If the brain is affected, they may have headaches, vomiting, confusion, loss of muscle control, or seizures. Leukemia also can affect other parts of the body such as the digestive tract, kidneys, lungs, heart, or testes.

Common symptoms of chronic or acute leukemia may include the following:

- Swollen lymph nodes that usually don't hurt (especially lymph nodes in the neck or armpit)

- Fevers or night sweats

- Frequent infections

- Feeling weak or tired

- Bleeding and bruising easily (bleeding gums, purplish patches in the skin, or tiny red spots under the skin)

- Swelling or discomfort in the abdomen (from a swollen spleen or liver)

- Weight loss for no known reason

- Pain in the bones or joints

Most often, these symptoms are not due to cancer. An infection or other health problems may also cause these symptoms. Only a doctor can tell for sure.

Treatment

People with leukemia have many treatment options. The options are watchful waiting, chemotherapy, targeted therapy, biological therapy, radiation therapy, and stem cell transplant. If your spleen is enlarged, your doctor may suggest surgery to remove it. Sometimes a combination of these treatments is used.

The choice of treatment depends mainly on the type of leukemia (acute or chronic), your age, and whether leukemia cells were found in your cerebrospinal fluid. It also may depend on certain features of the leukemia cells. Your doctor also considers your symptoms and general health.

People with acute leukemia need to be treated right away. The goal of treatment is to destroy signs of leukemia in the body and make symptoms go away. This is called a remission. After people go into remission, more therapy may be given to prevent a relapse. This type of therapy is called consolidation therapy or maintenance therapy. Many people with acute leukemia can be cured.

If you have chronic leukemia without symptoms, you may not need cancer treatment right away. Your doctor will watch your health closely so that treatment can start when you begin to have symptoms. Not getting cancer treatment right away is called watchful waiting.

Chemotherapy

Many people with leukemia are treated with chemotherapy. Chemotherapy uses drugs to destroy leukemia cells. Depending on the type of leukemia, you may receive a single drug or a combination of two or more drugs. You may receive chemotherapy by mouth, into a vein (IV), through a catheter (a thin, flexible tube), or into the cerebrospinal fluid (into the spinal fluid or under the scalp).

Chemotherapy is usually given in cycles. Each cycle has a treatment period followed by a rest period. You may have your treatment in a clinic, at the doctor's office, or at home. Some people may need to stay in the hospital for treatment. The side effects depend mainly on which drugs are given and how much. Chemotherapy kills fast-growing leukemia cells, but the drug can also harm normal cells that divide rapidly, including blood cells, cells in hair roots, cells that line the digestive tract, and sperm or egg cells.

Targeted Therapy

People with chronic myeloid leukemia and some with acute lymphoblastic leukemia may receive drugs called targeted therapy. Targeted therapies use drugs that block the growth of leukemia cells. For example, a targeted therapy may block the action of an abnormal protein that stimulates the growth of leukemia cells.

Side effects include swelling, bloating, and sudden weight gain. Targeted therapy can also cause anemia, nausea, vomiting, diarrhea, muscle cramps, or a rash.

Biological Therapy

Some people with leukemia receive drugs called biological therapy. Biological therapy for leukemia is treatment that improves the body's natural defenses against the disease.

The side effects of biological therapy differ with the types of substances used, and from person to person. Biological therapies commonly cause a rash or swelling where the drug is injected. They also may cause a headache, muscle aches, a fever, or weakness. Your health care team may check your blood for signs of anemia and other problems.

Radiation Therapy

Radiation therapy (also called radiotherapy) uses high-energy rays to kill leukemia cells. People receive radiation therapy at a hospital or clinic.

The side effects of radiation therapy depend mainly on the dose of radiation and the part of the body that is treated. For example, radiation to your abdomen can cause nausea, vomiting, and diarrhea. In addition, your skin in the area being treated may become red, dry, and tender. You also may lose your hair in the treated area.

You are likely to be very tired during radiation therapy, especially after several weeks of treatment. Resting is important, but doctors usually advise patients to try to stay as active as they can.

Although the side effects of radiation therapy can be distressing, they can usually be treated or controlled. It may also help to know that, in most cases, the side effects are not permanent. However, you may want to discuss with your doctor the possible long-term effects of radiation treatment.

Stem Cell Transplant

Some people with leukemia receive a stem cell transplant. A stem cell transplant allows you to be treated with high doses of drugs, radiation, or both. The high doses destroy both leukemia cells and normal blood cells in the bone marrow. After you receive high-dose chemotherapy, radiation therapy, or both, you receive healthy stem cells through a large vein. (It's like getting a blood transfusion.) New blood cells develop from the transplanted stem cells. The new blood cells replace the ones that were destroyed by treatment.

Stem cell transplants take place in the hospital. Stem cells may come from you or from someone who donates their stem cells to you.

After a stem cell transplant, you may stay in the hospital for several weeks or months. You'll be at risk for infections and bleeding because of the large doses of chemotherapy or radiation you received. In time, the transplanted stem cells will begin to produce healthy blood cells.

Supportive Care

Supportive care is treatment to prevent or fight infections, to control pain and other symptoms, to relieve the side effects of therapy, and to help you cope with the feelings that a diagnosis of cancer can bring. You may receive supportive care to prevent or control these problems and to improve your comfort and quality of life during treatment.

- **Infections:** Because people with leukemia get infections very easily, you may receive antibiotics and other drugs.
- **Anemia And Bleeding:** Anemia and bleeding are other problems that often require supportive care. You may need a transfusion of red blood cells or platelets. Transfusions help treat anemia and reduce the risk of serious bleeding.
- **Dental Problems:** Leukemia and chemotherapy can make the mouth sensitive, easily infected, and likely to bleed.

Nutrition And Physical Activity

It's important for you to take care of yourself by eating well and staying as active as you can. You need the right amount of calories to maintain a good weight. You also need enough protein to keep up your strength. Eating well may help you feel better and have more energy.

Sometimes, especially during or soon after treatment, you may not feel like eating. You may be uncomfortable or tired. You may find that foods do not taste as good as they used to. In addition, the side effects of treatment (such as poor appetite, nausea, vomiting, or mouth sores) can make it hard to eat well. Your doctor, a registered dietitian, or another health care provider can suggest ways to deal with these problems.

Research shows that people with cancer feel better when they are active. Walking, yoga, and other activities can keep you strong and increase your energy. Exercise may reduce nausea and pain and make treatment easier to handle. It also can help relieve stress. Whatever physical activity you choose, be sure to talk to your doctor before you start. Also, if your activity causes you pain or other problems, be sure to let your doctor or nurse know about it.

Follow-Up Care

You'll need regular checkups after treatment for leukemia. Checkups help ensure that any changes in your health are noted and treated if needed. If you have any health problems between checkups, you should contact your doctor.

Your doctor will check for return of the cancer. Even when the cancer seems to be completely destroyed, the disease sometimes returns because undetected leukemia cells remained somewhere in your body after treatment. Also, checkups help detect health problems that can result from cancer treatment.

Checkups may include a careful physical exam, blood tests, cytogenetics, x-rays, bone marrow aspiration, or spinal tap.

Chapter 29

Lung Cancer

The Lungs

Your lungs are a pair of large organs in your chest. They are part of your respiratory system. Air enters your body through your nose or mouth. It passes through your windpipe (trachea) and through each bronchus, and goes into your lungs. When you breathe in, your lungs expand with air. This is how your body gets oxygen. When you breathe out, air goes out of your lungs. This is how your body gets rid of carbon dioxide.

Risk Factors

Doctors cannot always explain why one person develops lung cancer and another does not. However, we do know that a person with certain risk factors may be more likely than others to develop lung cancer. A risk factor is something that may increase the chance of developing a disease.

Studies have found the following risk factors for lung cancer:

Tobacco Smoke: Tobacco smoke causes most cases of lung cancer. It's by far the most important risk factor for lung cancer. Harmful substances in smoke

About This Chapter: This chapter includes excerpts from "What You Need to Know about Lung Cancer," National Cancer Institute, July 26, 2007; and PDQ® Cancer Information Summary. National Cancer Institute; Bethesda, MD. Lung Cancer Prevention (PDQ®): Patient Version. Updated 02/2006. Available at: http://cancergov. Accessed August 21, 2009.

damage lung cells. That's why smoking cigarettes, pipes, or cigars can cause lung cancer and why secondhand smoke can cause lung cancer in nonsmokers. The more a person is exposed to smoke, the greater the risk of lung cancer.

Radon: Radon is a radioactive gas that you cannot see, smell, or taste. It forms in soil and rocks. People who work in mines may be exposed to radon. In some parts of the country, radon is found in houses. Radon damages lung cells, and people exposed to radon are at increased risk of lung cancer. The risk of lung cancer from radon is even higher for smokers.

Asbestos And Other Substances: People who have certain jobs (such as those who work in the construction and chemical industries) have an increased risk of lung cancer. Exposure to asbestos, arsenic, chromium, nickel, soot, tar, and other substances can cause lung cancer. The risk is highest for those with years of exposure. The risk of lung cancer from these substances is even higher for smokers.

Air Pollution: Air pollution may slightly increase the risk of lung cancer. The risk from air pollution is higher for smokers.

Family History: People with a father, mother, brother, or sister who had lung cancer may be at slightly increased risk of the disease, even if they don't smoke.

Personal History: People who have had lung cancer are at increased risk of developing a second lung tumor.

Age: Most people are older than 65 years when diagnosed with lung cancer.

Researchers have studied other possible risk factors. For example, having certain lung diseases (such as tuberculosis or bronchitis) for many years may increase the risk of lung cancer. It's not yet clear whether having certain lung diseases is a risk factor for lung cancer.

How To Quit Smoking

Quitting is important for anyone who smokes tobacco—even people who have smoked for many years. For people who already have cancer, quitting may reduce the chance of getting another cancer. Quitting also can help cancer treatments work better.

> ### ❖ It's A Fact!!
>
> The most important risk factor for lung cancer is smoke from cigarettes, pipes, and cigars or from secondhand smoke. Smoking also increases the risks associated with other risk factors such as exposure to radon, air pollution, asbestos, arsenic, chromium, nickel, soot, and tar.
>
> Source: National Cancer Institute, July 26, 2007.

Screening

Currently, there is no generally accepted screening test for lung cancer. Several methods of detecting lung cancer have been studied as possible screening tests. The methods under study include tests of sputum (mucus brought up from the lungs by coughing), chest x-rays, or spiral (helical) CT scans.

However, screening tests have risks. For example, an abnormal x-ray result could lead to other procedures (such as surgery to check for cancer cells), but a person with an abnormal test result might not have lung cancer. Studies so far have not shown that screening tests lower the number of deaths from lung cancer.

Symptoms

Early lung cancer often does not cause symptoms. But as the cancer grows, common symptoms may include the following:

- A cough that gets worse or does not go away
- Breathing trouble, such as shortness of breath
- Constant chest pain
- Coughing up blood
- A hoarse voice
- Frequent lung infections, such as pneumonia
- Feeling very tired all the time
- Weight loss with no known cause

Most often these symptoms are not due to cancer. Other health problems can cause some of these symptoms. Anyone with such symptoms should see a doctor to be diagnosed and treated as early as possible.

Diagnosis

If you have a symptom that suggests lung cancer, your doctor must find out whether it's from cancer or something else. Your doctor may ask about your personal and family medical history. Your doctor may order blood tests, and you may have one or more of the following tests:

- **Physical Exam:** Your doctor checks for general signs of health, listens to your breathing, and checks for fluid in the lungs. Your doctor may feel for swollen lymph nodes and a swollen liver.

- **Chest X-Ray:** X-ray pictures of your chest may show tumors or abnormal fluid.

- **CT Scan:** Doctors often use CT scans to take pictures of tissue inside the chest. An x-ray machine linked to a computer takes several pictures. For a spiral CT scan, the CT scanner rotates around you as you lie on a table. The table passes through the center of the scanner. The pictures may show a tumor, abnormal fluid, or swollen lymph nodes.

✔ Quick Tip

There are many ways to get help quitting smoking:

- Ask your doctor about medicine or nicotine replacement therapy, such as a patch, gum, lozenge, nasal spray, or inhaler. Your doctor can suggest a number of treatments that help people quit.

- Ask your doctor to help you find local programs or trained professionals who help people stop using tobacco.

- Call staff at NCI's Smoking Quitline (877-44U-QUIT) or instant message them through LiveHelp.

- Go online to Smokefree.gov (http://www.smokefree.gov), a federal government website. It offers a guide to quitting smoking and a list of other resources.

Source: National Cancer Institute, July 26, 2007.

❖ It's A Fact!!

Lung Cancer Is The Leading Cause Of Cancer Deaths In U.S. Men And Women

Lung cancer can often be associated with known risk factors for the disease. Many risk factors can be changed, but not all can be avoided.

Studies show that smoking tobacco products in any form is the major cause of lung cancer. People who stop smoking and never start again lower their risk of developing lung cancer or of having lung cancer recur (come back). Many products, such as nicotine gum, nicotine sprays, nicotine inhalers, nicotine patches, or nicotine lozenges, as well as antidepressant drugs, may be helpful to people trying to quit smoking. Never smoking lowers the risk of dying from lung cancer.

Secondhand tobacco smoke also causes lung cancer. This is smoke that comes from a burning cigarette or other tobacco product, or smoke that is exhaled by smokers. People who inhale secondhand smoke are exposed to the same cancer-causing agents as smokers, although in weaker amounts. Inhaling secondhand smoke is called involuntary or passive smoking.

There are other causes of lung cancer in the environment, but their effect on lung cancer rates is small compared to the effect of cigarette smoking.

Source: Excerpted from "Lung Cancer Prevention (PDQ), Patient Version," National Cancer Institute (www.cancer.gov), February 16, 2006.

The only sure way to know if lung cancer is present is for a pathologist to check samples of cells or tissue. The pathologist studies the sample under a microscope and performs other tests. Your doctor may order one or more of the following tests to collect samples:

- **Sputum Cytology:** Thick fluid (sputum) is coughed up from the lungs. The lab checks samples of sputum for cancer cells.

- **Thoracentesis:** The doctor uses a long needle to remove fluid (pleural fluid) from the chest. The lab checks the fluid for cancer cells.

- **Bronchoscopy:** The doctor inserts a thin, lighted tube (a bronchoscope) through the nose or mouth into the lung. This allows an exam of the lungs and the air passages that lead to them. The doctor may take a sample of cells with a needle, brush, or other tool. The doctor also may wash the area with water to collect cells in the water.

- **Fine-Needle Aspiration:** The doctor uses a thin needle to remove tissue or fluid from the lung or lymph node. Sometimes the doctor uses a CT scan or other imaging method to guide the needle to a lung tumor or lymph node.

- **Thoracoscopy:** The surgeon makes several small incisions in your chest and back. The surgeon looks at the lungs and nearby tissues with a thin, lighted tube. If an abnormal area is seen, a biopsy to check for cancer cells may be needed.

- **Thoracotomy:** The surgeon opens the chest with a long incision. Lymph nodes and other tissue may be removed.

- **Mediastinoscopy:** The surgeon makes an incision at the top of the breastbone. A thin, lighted tube is used to see inside the chest. The surgeon may take tissue and lymph node samples.

Types Of Lung Cancer

The pathologist checks the samples for cancer cells. If cancer is found, the pathologist reports the type. The types of lung cancer are treated differently. The most common types are named for how the lung cancer cells look under a microscope:

- **Small Cell Lung Cancer:** About 13% of lung cancers are small cell lung cancers. This type tends to spread quickly.

- **Non-Small Cell Lung Cancer:** Most lung cancers (about 87%) are non-small cell lung cancers. This type spreads more slowly than small cell lung cancer.

Staging

To plan the best treatment, your doctor needs to know the type of lung cancer and the extent (stage) of the disease. Staging is a careful attempt to find out whether the cancer has spread, and if so, to what parts of the body. Lung cancer spreads most often to the lymph nodes, brain, bones, liver, and adrenal glands.

When cancer spreads from its original place to another part of the body, the new tumor has the same kind of cancer cells and the same name as the original cancer. For example, if lung cancer spreads to the liver, the cancer cells in the liver are actually lung cancer cells. The disease is metastatic lung cancer, not liver cancer. For that reason, it's treated as lung cancer, not liver cancer. Doctors call the new tumor "distant" or metastatic disease.

Treatment

Your doctor may refer you to a specialist who has experience treating lung cancer, or you may ask for a referral. You may have a team of specialists. Specialists who treat lung cancer include thoracic (chest) surgeons, thoracic surgical oncologists, medical oncologists, and radiation oncologists. Your health care team may also include a pulmonologist (a lung specialist), a respiratory therapist, an oncology nurse, and a registered dietitian.

Lung cancer is hard to control with current treatments. For that reason, many doctors encourage patients with this disease to consider taking part in a clinical trial. Clinical trials are an important option for people with all stages of lung cancer.

The choice of treatment depends mainly on the type of lung cancer and its stage. People with lung cancer may have surgery, chemotherapy, radiation therapy, targeted therapy, or a combination of treatments.

People with limited stage small cell lung cancer usually have radiation therapy and chemotherapy. For a very small lung tumor, a person may have surgery and chemotherapy. Most people with extensive stage small cell lung cancer are treated with chemotherapy only.

People with non-small cell lung cancer may have surgery, chemotherapy, radiation therapy, or a combination of treatments. The treatment choices are different for each stage. Some people with advanced cancer receive targeted therapy.

Surgery

Surgery for lung cancer removes the tissue that contains the tumor. The surgeon removes part or all of the lung. The surgeon also removes nearby lymph nodes.

✎ **What's It Mean?**

Wedge Resection (Segmentectomy): The surgeon removes the tumor and a small part of the lung.

Lobectomy (Sleeve Lobectomy): The surgeon removes a lobe of the lung. This is the most common surgery for lung cancer.

Pneumonectomy: The surgeon removes the entire lung.

Source: National Cancer Institute, July 26, 2007.

After lung surgery, air and fluid collect in the chest. A chest tube allows the fluid to drain. Also, a nurse or respiratory therapist will teach you coughing and breathing exercises. You'll need to do the exercises several times a day.

The time it takes to heal after surgery is different for everyone. Your hospital stay may be a week or longer. It may be several weeks before you return to normal activities.

Medicine can help control your pain after surgery. Before surgery, you should discuss the plan for pain relief with your doctor or nurse. After surgery, your doctor can adjust the plan if you need more pain relief.

Radiation Therapy

Radiation therapy (also called radiotherapy) uses high-energy rays to kill cancer cells. It affects cells only in the treated area.

You may receive external radiation. This is the most common type of radiation therapy for lung cancer. The radiation comes from a large machine outside your body. Most people go to a hospital or clinic for treatment. Treatments are usually five days a week for several weeks.

Another type of radiation therapy is internal radiation (brachytherapy). Internal radiation is seldom used for people with lung cancer. The radiation comes from a seed, wire, or another device put inside your body.

The side effects depend mainly on the type of radiation therapy, the dose of radiation, and the part of your body that is treated. External radiation therapy to the chest may harm the esophagus, causing problems with swallowing. You may also feel very tired. In addition, your skin in the treated area may become red, dry, and tender. After internal radiation therapy, a person may cough up small amounts of blood. Your doctor can suggest ways to ease these problems.

Chemotherapy

Chemotherapy uses anticancer drugs to kill cancer cells. Anticancer drugs for lung cancer are usually given through a vein (intravenous). Some anticancer drugs can be taken by mouth.

Chemotherapy is given in cycles. You have a rest period after each treatment period. The length of the rest period and the number of cycles depend on the anticancer drugs used.

The side effects depend mainly on which drugs are given and how much. The drugs can harm normal cells that divide rapidly. Some drugs for lung cancer can cause hearing loss, joint pain, and tingling or numbness in your hands and feet. These side effects usually go away after treatment ends.

When radiation therapy and chemotherapy are given at the same time, the side effects may be worse.

Targeted Therapy

Targeted therapy uses drugs to block the growth and spread of cancer cells. Some people with non-small cell lung cancer that has spread receive targeted therapy.

There are two kinds of targeted therapy for lung cancer. One kind is given through a vein (intravenous) at the doctor's office, hospital, or clinic. It's given at the same time as chemotherapy. The side effects may include bleeding, coughing up blood, a rash, high blood pressure, abdominal pain, vomiting, or diarrhea.

Another kind of targeted therapy is taken by mouth. It isn't given with chemotherapy. The side effects may include rash, diarrhea, and shortness of breath.

Follow-Up Care

You'll need regular checkups after treatment for lung cancer. Even when there are no longer any signs of cancer, the disease sometimes returns because undetected cancer cells remained somewhere in your body after treatment.

Checkups help ensure that any changes in your health are noted and treated if needed. Checkups may include a physical exam, blood tests, chest x-rays, CT scans, and bronchoscopy.

Chapter 30

Oral Cancer

The Mouth And Throat

This chapter is about cancers that occur in the mouth (oral cavity) and the part of the throat at the back of the mouth (oropharynx). The oral cavity and oropharynx have many parts:

- Lips
- Lining of your cheeks
- Salivary glands (glands that make saliva)
- Roof of your mouth (hard palate)
- Back of your mouth (soft palate and uvula)
- Floor of your mouth (area under the tongue)
- Gums and teeth
- Tongue
- Tonsils

Oral cancer is part of a group of cancers called head and neck cancers. Oral cancer can develop in any part of the oral cavity or oropharynx. Most oral cancers begin in the tongue and in the floor of the mouth. Almost all oral

About This Chapter: Text in this chapter is excerpted from "What You Need to Know about Oral Cancer," National Cancer Institute, September 8, 2004.

cancers begin in the flat cells (squamous cells) that cover the surfaces of the mouth, tongue, and lips. These cancers are called squamous cell carcinomas.

When oral cancer spreads (metastasizes), it usually travels through the lymphatic system. Cancer cells that enter the lymphatic system are carried along by lymph, a clear, watery fluid. The cancer cells often appear first in nearby lymph nodes in the neck.

Cancer cells can also spread to other parts of the neck, the lungs, and other parts of the body.

Who's At Risk For Oral Cancer?

Research has shown that people with certain risk factors are more likely than others to develop oral cancer. A risk factor is anything that increases your chance of developing a disease. The following are risk factors for oral cancer:

- **Tobacco:** Smoking cigarettes, cigars, or pipes; using chewing tobacco; and dipping snuff are all linked to oral cancer. The use of other tobacco products (such as bidis and kreteks) may also increase the risk of oral cancer. Heavy smokers who use tobacco for a long time are most at risk. The risk is even higher for tobacco users who drink alcohol heavily. In fact, three out of four oral cancers occur in people who use alcohol, tobacco, or both alcohol and tobacco.

- **Alcohol:** People who drink alcohol are more likely to develop oral cancer than people who don't drink. The risk increases with the amount of alcohol that a person consumes. The risk increases even more if the person both drinks alcohol and uses tobacco.

♣ It's A Fact!!
Tobacco use accounts for most oral cancers. Quitting tobacco reduces the risk of oral cancer. Also, quitting reduces the chance that a person with oral cancer will get a second cancer in the head and neck region. People who stop smoking can also reduce their risk of cancer of the lung, larynx, mouth, pancreas, bladder, and esophagus.

✤ It's A Fact!!

Not using tobacco may be the most important thing you can do to prevent oral cancers. There are many resources to help smokers quit:

- Groups offer counseling in person or by telephone.
- Your doctor or dentist can help you find a local smoking cessation program.
- Your doctor can tell you about medicine (bupropion) or about nicotine replacement therapy, which comes as a patch, gum, lozenges, nasal spray, or inhaler.

- **Sun:** Cancer of the lip can be caused by exposure to the sun. Using a lotion or lip balm that has a sunscreen can reduce the risk. Wearing a hat with a brim can also block the sun's harmful rays. The risk of cancer of the lip increases if the person also smokes.

- **Personal History:** People who have had head and neck cancer are at increased risk of developing another primary head and neck cancer. Smoking increases this risk.

Some studies suggest that not eating enough fruits and vegetables may increase the chance of getting oral cancer. Scientists also are studying whether infections with certain viruses (such as the human papillomavirus) are linked to oral cancer.

Early Detection

Your regular checkup is a good time for your dentist or doctor to check your entire mouth for signs of cancer. Regular checkups can detect the early stages of oral cancer or conditions that may lead to oral cancer. Ask your doctor or dentist about checking the tissues in your mouth as part of your routine exam.

Common symptoms of oral cancer include:

- Patches inside your mouth or on your lips that are white, a mixture of red and white, or red

- White patches (leukoplakia) are the most common and sometimes become malignant

- Mixed red and white patches (erythroleukoplakia) are more likely than white patches to become malignant

- Red patches (erythroplakia) are brightly colored, smooth areas that often become malignant

- A sore on your lip or in your mouth that won't heal

- Bleeding in your mouth

- Loose teeth

- Difficulty or pain when swallowing

- Difficulty wearing dentures

- A lump in your neck

- An earache

Anyone with these symptoms should see a doctor or dentist so that any problem can be diagnosed and treated as early as possible. Most often, these symptoms do not mean cancer. An infection or another problem can cause the same symptoms.

Diagnosis

If you have symptoms that suggest oral cancer, the doctor or dentist checks your mouth and throat for red or white patches, lumps, swelling, or other problems. This exam includes looking carefully at the roof of the mouth, back of the throat, and insides of the cheeks and lips. The doctor or dentist also gently pulls out your tongue so it can be checked on the sides and underneath. The floor of your mouth and lymph nodes in your neck also are checked.

If an exam shows an abnormal area, a small sample of tissue may be removed. Removing tissue to look for cancer cells is called a biopsy. Usually, a biopsy is done with local anesthesia. Sometimes, it is done under general anesthesia. A pathologist then looks at the tissue under a microscope to check for cancer cells. A biopsy is the only sure way to know if the abnormal area is cancerous.

Staging

If the biopsy shows that cancer is present, your doctor needs to know the stage (extent) of your disease to plan the best treatment. The stage is based on the size of the tumor, whether the cancer has spread and, if so, to what parts of the body.

Staging may require lab tests. It also may involve endoscopy and the doctor may also order one or more imaging tests to learn whether the cancer has spread.

Treatment

Your doctor may refer you to a specialist. Specialists who treat oral cancer include oral and maxillofacial surgeons, otolaryngologists (ear, nose, and throat doctors), medical oncologists, radiation oncologists, and plastic surgeons. You may be referred to a team that includes specialists in surgery, radiation therapy, or chemotherapy. Other health care professionals who may work with the specialists as a team include a dentist, speech pathologist, nutritionist, and mental health counselor.

The choice of treatment depends mainly on your general health, where in your mouth or oropharynx the cancer began, the size of the tumor, and whether the cancer has spread. Oral cancer treatment may include surgery, radiation therapy, or chemotherapy. Some patients have a combination of treatments.

At any stage of disease, people with oral cancer may have treatment to control pain and other symptoms, to relieve the side effects of therapy, and to ease emotional and practical problems. This kind of treatment is called supportive care, symptom management, or palliative care.

You may want to talk to the doctor about taking part in a clinical trial, a research study of new treatment methods.

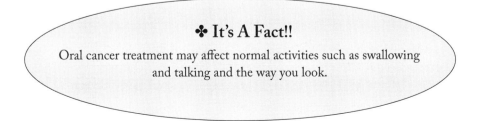

✤ It's A Fact!!
Oral cancer treatment may affect normal activities such as swallowing and talking and the way you look.

Surgery

Surgery to remove the tumor in the mouth or throat is a common treatment for oral cancer. Sometimes the surgeon also removes lymph nodes in the neck. Other tissues in the mouth and neck may be removed as well. Patients may have surgery alone or in combination with radiation therapy.

Radiation Therapy

Radiation therapy (also called radiotherapy) uses high-energy rays to kill cancer cells. Doctors use two types of radiation therapy to treat oral cancer, external radiation and internal radiation.

- **External Radiation:** The radiation comes from a machine. Patients go to the hospital or clinic once or twice a day, generally five days a week for several weeks.

- **Internal Radiation (Implant Radiation):** The radiation comes from radioactive material placed in seeds, needles, or thin plastic tubes put directly in the tissue. The patient stays in the hospital. The implants remain in place for several days. Usually they are removed before the patient goes home.

Some people with oral cancer have both kinds of radiation therapy.

Chemotherapy

Chemotherapy uses anticancer drugs to kill cancer cells. It is called systemic therapy because it enters the bloodstream and can affect cancer cells throughout the body.

Chemotherapy is usually given by injection. It may be given in an outpatient part of the hospital, at the doctor's office, or at home. Rarely, a hospital stay may be needed.

Nutrition

Eating well during cancer treatment means getting enough calories and protein to prevent weight loss, regain strength, and rebuild healthy tissues. But eating well may be difficult after treatment for oral cancer. Some people with cancer find it hard to eat because they lose their appetite. They may not feel like eating because they are uncomfortable or tired. A dry or sore mouth or changes in smell and taste also may make eating difficult.

✦ **It's A Fact!!**

People who have had oral cancer have a chance of developing a new cancer in the mouth, throat, or other areas of the head and neck. This is especially true for those who use tobacco or who drink alcohol heavily. Doctors strongly urge their patients to stop using tobacco and drinking to cut down the risk of a new cancer and other health problems.

If your mouth is dry, you may find that soft foods moistened with sauces or gravies are easier to eat. Thick soups, puddings, and milkshakes often are easier to swallow. Nurses and dietitians can help you choose the right foods.

After surgery or radiation therapy for oral cancer, some people need a feeding tube. In almost all cases, the tube is temporary. Most people gradually return to a regular diet.

Reconstruction

Some people with oral cancer may need to have plastic or reconstructive surgery to rebuild the bones or tissues of the mouth. Research has led to many advances in the way bones and tissues can be replaced.

Some people may need dental implants. Or they may need to have grafts (tissue moved from another part of the body). Skin, muscle, and bone can be moved to the oral cavity from the chest, arm, or leg. The plastic surgeon uses this tissue for repair.

Rehabilitation

The health care team will help you return to normal activities as soon as possible. The goals of rehabilitation depend on the extent of the disease and type of treatment. Rehabilitation may include being fitted with a dental prosthesis (an artificial dental device) and having dental implants. It also may involve speech therapy, dietary counseling, or other services.

Follow-Up Care

Follow-up care after treatment for oral cancer is important. Even when the cancer seems to have been completely removed or destroyed, the disease sometimes returns because undetected cancer cells remained in the body after treatment. The doctor monitors your recovery and checks for recurrence of cancer. Checkups help ensure that any changes in your health are noted. Your doctor will probably encourage you to inspect your mouth regularly and continue to have exams when you visit your dentist. It is important to report any changes in your mouth right away.

Checkups include exams of the mouth, throat, and neck. From time to time, your doctor may do a complete physical exam, order blood tests, and take x-rays.

Chapter 31

Pancreatic Cancer

The Pancreas

The pancreas is a gland located deep in the abdomen between the stomach and the spine (backbone). The liver, intestine, and other organs surround the pancreas. The pancreas is about six inches long and is shaped like a flat pear. The widest part of the pancreas is the head, the middle section is the body, and the thinnest part is the tail.

The pancreas makes insulin and other hormones. These hormones enter the bloodstream and travel throughout the body. They help the body use or store the energy that comes from food. For example, insulin helps control the amount of sugar in the blood.

The pancreas also makes pancreatic juices. These juices contain enzymes that help digest food. The pancreas releases the juices into a system of ducts leading to the common bile duct. The common bile duct empties into the duodenum, the first section of the small intestine.

Most pancreatic cancers begin in the ducts that carry pancreatic juices. Cancer of the pancreas may be called pancreatic cancer or carcinoma of the pancreas.

About This Chapter: Text in this chapter is excerpted from "What You Need to Know about Cancer of the Pancreas," National Cancer Institute, September 19, 2002.

A rare type of pancreatic cancer begins in the cells that make insulin and other hormones. Cancer that begins in these cells is called islet cell cancer. This chapter does not deal with this rare disease.

When cancer of the pancreas spreads (metastasizes) outside the pancreas, cancer cells are often found in nearby lymph nodes. If the cancer has reached these nodes, it means that cancer cells may have spread to other lymph nodes or other tissues, such as the liver or lungs. Sometimes cancer of the pancreas spreads to the peritoneum, the tissue that lines the abdomen.

When cancer spreads from its original place to another part of the body, the new tumor has the same kind of abnormal cells and the same name as the primary tumor. For example, if cancer of the pancreas spreads to the liver, the cancer cells in the liver are pancreatic cancer cells. The disease is metastatic pancreatic cancer, not liver cancer. It is treated as pancreatic cancer, not liver cancer.

Who's At Risk For Pancreatic Cancer?

No one knows the exact causes of pancreatic cancer. Research has shown that people with certain risk factors are more likely than others to develop pancreatic cancer. Studies have found the following risk factors:

- **Age:** The likelihood of developing pancreatic cancer increases with age. Most pancreatic cancers occur in people over the age of 60.

- **Smoking:** Cigarette smokers are two or three times more likely than nonsmokers to develop pancreatic cancer.

- **Diabetes:** Pancreatic cancer occurs more often in people who have diabetes than in people who do not.

- **Gender:** More men than women are diagnosed with pancreatic cancer.

- **Race:** African Americans are more likely than Asians, Hispanics, or whites to get pancreatic cancer.

- **Family History:** The risk for developing pancreatic cancer triples if a person's mother, father, sister, or brother had the disease. Also, a family history of colon or ovarian cancer increases the risk of pancreatic cancer.

- **Chronic Pancreatitis:** Chronic pancreatitis is a painful condition of the pancreas. Some evidence suggests that chronic pancreatitis may increase the risk of pancreatic cancer.

Other studies suggest that exposure to certain chemicals in the workplace or a diet high in fat may increase the chance of getting pancreatic cancer.

Most people with known risk factors do not get pancreatic cancer. On the other hand, many who do get the disease have none of these factors.

Symptoms

Pancreatic cancer is sometimes called a "silent disease" because early pancreatic cancer often does not cause symptoms. But, as the cancer grows, symptoms may include the following:

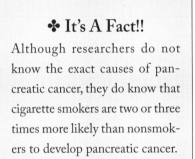

❖ It's A Fact!!

Although researchers do not know the exact causes of pancreatic cancer, they do know that cigarette smokers are two or three times more likely than nonsmokers to develop pancreatic cancer.

- Pain in the upper abdomen or upper back

- Yellow skin and eyes, and dark urine from jaundice

- Weakness

- Loss of appetite

- Nausea and vomiting

- Weight loss

These symptoms are not sure signs of pancreatic cancer. An infection or other problem could also cause these symptoms. Only a doctor can diagnose the cause of a person's symptoms. Anyone with these symptoms should see a doctor so that the doctor can treat any problem as early as possible.

Diagnosis

If a patient has symptoms that suggest pancreatic cancer, the doctor asks about the patient's medical history. The doctor may perform a number of procedures, including one or more of the following:

- **Physical Exam:** The doctor examines the skin and eyes for signs of jaundice. The doctor then feels the abdomen to check for changes in the area near the pancreas, liver, and gallbladder. The doctor also checks for ascites, an abnormal buildup of fluid in the abdomen.

- **Lab Tests:** The doctor may take blood, urine, and stool samples to check for bilirubin and other substances. Bilirubin is a substance that passes from the liver to the gallbladder to the intestine. If the common bile duct is blocked by a tumor, the bilirubin cannot pass through normally. Blockage may cause the level of bilirubin in the blood, stool, or urine to become very high. High bilirubin levels can result from cancer or from noncancerous conditions.

- **CT Scan (Computed Tomography):** An x-ray machine linked to a computer takes a series of detailed pictures.

- **Ultrasonography:** The ultrasound device uses sound waves that cannot be heard by humans. The sound waves produce a pattern of echoes as they bounce off internal organs. The echoes create a picture of the pancreas and other organs inside the abdomen. The echoes from tumors are different from echoes made by healthy tissues. The ultrasound procedure may use an external or internal device, or both types. Transabdominal ultrasound is external. To make images of the pancreas, the doctor places the ultrasound device on the abdomen and slowly moves it around. Endoscopic ultrasound (EUS) is internal. The doctor passes a thin, lighted tube (endoscope) through the patient's mouth and stomach, down into the first part of the small intestine. At the tip of the endoscope is an ultrasound device. The doctor slowly withdraws the endoscope from the intestine toward the stomach to make images of the pancreas and surrounding organs and tissues.

- **Endoscopic Retrograde Cholangiopancreatography (ERCP):** The doctor passes an endoscope through the patient's mouth and stomach, down into the first part of the small intestine. The doctor slips a smaller tube (catheter) through the endoscope into the bile ducts and pancreatic ducts. After injecting dye through the catheter into the ducts, the doctor takes x-ray pictures. The x-rays can show whether the ducts are narrowed or blocked by a tumor or other condition.

- **Percutaneous Transhepatic Cholangiography (PTC):** A dye is injected through a thin needle inserted through the skin into the liver. Unless there is a blockage, the dye should move freely through the bile ducts. The dye makes the bile ducts show up on x-ray pictures. From the pictures, the doctor can tell whether there is a blockage from a tumor or other condition.

- **Biopsy:** In some cases, the doctor may remove tissue. A pathologist then uses a microscope to look for cancer cells in the tissue. The doctor may obtain tissue in several ways. One way is by inserting a needle into the pancreas to remove cells. This is called fine-needle aspiration. The doctor uses x-ray or ultrasound to guide the needle. Sometimes the doctor obtains a sample of tissue during EUS or ERCP. Another way is to open the abdomen during an operation.

Staging

When pancreatic cancer is diagnosed, the doctor needs to know the stage, or extent, of the disease to plan the best treatment. Staging is a careful attempt to find out the size of the tumor in the pancreas, whether the cancer has spread, and if so, to what parts of the body.

The doctor may determine the stage of pancreatic cancer at the time of diagnosis, or the patient may need to have more tests. Such tests may include blood tests, a CT scan, ultrasonography, laparoscopy, or angiography. The test results will help the doctor decide which treatment is appropriate.

Treatment

Cancer of the pancreas is very hard to control with current treatments. For that reason, many doctors encourage patients with this disease to consider taking part in a clinical trial. Clinical trials are an important option for people with all stages of pancreatic cancer.

At this time, pancreatic cancer can be cured only when it is found at an early stage, before it has spread. However, other treatments may be able to control the disease and help patients live longer and feel better. When a cure or control of the disease is not possible, some patients and their doctors choose palliative therapy. Palliative therapy aims to improve quality of life by controlling pain and other problems caused by this disease.

The doctor may refer patients to an oncologist, a doctor who specializes in treating cancer. Specialists who treat pancreatic cancer include surgeons, medical oncologists, and radiation oncologists. Treatment depends on where in the pancreas the tumor started and whether the disease has spread. When planning treatment, the doctor also considers other factors, including the patient's age and general health.

Nutrition

People with pancreatic cancer may not feel like eating, especially if they are uncomfortable or tired. Also, the side effects of treatment such as poor appetite, nausea, or vomiting can make eating difficult. Foods may taste different. Nevertheless, patients should try to get enough calories and protein to control weight loss, maintain strength, and promote healing. Also, eating well often helps people with cancer feel better and have more energy.

Careful planning and checkups are important. Cancer of the pancreas and its treatment may make it hard for patients to digest food and maintain the proper blood sugar level. The doctor will check the patient for weight loss, weakness, and lack of energy. Patients may need to take medicines to replace the enzymes and hormones made by the pancreas. The doctor will watch the patient closely and adjust the doses of these medicines.

The doctor, dietitian, or other health care provider can advise patients about ways to maintain a healthy diet.

Follow-Up Care

Follow-up care after treatment for pancreatic cancer is an important part of the overall treatment plan. Patients should not hesitate to discuss follow-up care with their doctor. Regular checkups ensure that any changes in health are noticed. Any problem that develops can be found and treated. Checkups may include a physical exam, laboratory tests, and imaging procedures.

Chapter 32

Stomach Cancer

The Stomach

The stomach is part of the digestive system. It is a hollow organ in the upper abdomen, under the ribs. The wall of the stomach has five layers:

- **Inner Layer Or Lining (Mucosa):** Juices made by glands in the inner layer help digest food. Most stomach cancers begin in this layer.

- **Submucosa:** This is the support tissue for the inner layer.

- **Muscle Layer:** Muscles in this layer create a rippling motion that mixes and mashes food.

- **Subserosa:** This is the support tissue for the outer layer.

- **Outer Layer (Serosa):** The outer layer covers the stomach. It holds the stomach in place.

Food moves from the mouth through the esophagus to reach the stomach. In the stomach, the food becomes liquid. The liquid then moves into the small intestine, where it is digested even more.

Stomach cancer can affect nearby organs and lymph nodes:

About This Chapter: Text in this chapter is excerpted from "What You Need to Know about Stomach Cancer," National Cancer Institute, August 30, 2005.

- A stomach tumor can grow through the stomach's outer layer into nearby organs, such as the pancreas, esophagus, or intestine.

- Stomach cancer cells can spread through the blood to the liver, lungs, and other organs.

- Cancer cells also can spread through the lymphatic system to lymph nodes all over the body.

When cancer spreads from its original place to another part of the body, the new tumor has the same kind of abnormal cells and the same name as the original tumor. For example, if stomach cancer spreads to the liver, the cancer cells in the liver are actually stomach cancer cells. The disease is metastatic stomach cancer, not liver cancer. For that reason, it is treated as stomach cancer, not liver cancer. Doctors call the new tumor "distant" or metastatic disease.

Risk Factors

No one knows the exact causes of stomach cancer.

Research has shown that people with certain risk factors are more likely than others to develop stomach cancer. A risk factor is something that may increase the chance of developing a disease.

Studies have found the following risk factors for stomach cancer:

Age: Most people with this disease are 72 or older.

Sex: Men are more likely than women to develop stomach cancer.

Race: Stomach cancer is more common in Asian, Pacific Islander, Hispanic, and African Americans than in non-Hispanic white Americans.

Diet: Studies suggest that people who eat a diet high in foods that are smoked, salted, or pickled may be at increased risk for stomach cancer. On the other hand, eating fresh fruits and vegetables may protect against this disease.

Helicobacter pylori infection: *H. pylori* is a type of bacteria that commonly lives in the stomach. H. pylori infection increases the risk of stomach inflammation and stomach ulcers. It also increases the risk of stomach cancer, but only a small number of infected people develop stomach cancer. Although infection increases the risk, cancer is not contagious. You cannot catch stomach cancer from another person who has it.

Smoking: People who smoke are more likely to develop stomach cancer than people who do not smoke.

Health Problems: Conditions that cause inflammation or other problems in the stomach may increase the risk of stomach cancer:

- Stomach surgery
- Chronic gastritis (long-term inflammation of the stomach lining)
- Pernicious anemia (a blood disease that affects the stomach)

Family History: A rare type of stomach cancer runs in some families

Most people who have known risk factors do not develop stomach cancer. For example, many people have *H. pylori* in their stomach but never develop cancer. On the other hand, people who do develop the disease sometimes have no known risk factors.

Early stomach cancer often does not cause clear symptoms. As the cancer grows, the most common symptoms are discomfort in the stomach area, feeling full or bloated after a small meal, nausea and vomiting, and weight loss. Most often, these symptoms are not due to cancer. Other health problems, such as an ulcer or infection, can cause the same symptoms. Anyone with these symptoms should tell the doctor so that problems can be found and treated as early as possible.

❖ It's A Fact!!

Although doctors often cannot explain why one person develops stomach cancer and another does not, medical researchers do know that people who smoke are more likely to develop stomach cancer than people who do not smoke.

Diagnosis

If you have a symptom that suggests stomach cancer, your doctor must find out whether it is really due to cancer or to some other cause. Your doctor may refer you to a gastroenterologist, a doctor whose specialty is diagnosing and treating digestive problems.

The doctor asks about your personal and family health history. You may have blood or other lab tests such as the following:

- **Physical Exam:** The doctor checks your abdomen for fluid, swelling, or other changes. The doctor also feels for swollen lymph nodes. Your skin and eyes are checked to see if they seem yellow.

- **Upper GI Series:** The doctor orders x-rays of your esophagus and stomach. The x-rays are taken after you drink a barium solution. The solution makes your stomach show up more clearly on the x-rays.

- **Endoscopy:** The doctor uses a thin, lighted tube (endoscope) to look into your stomach. The doctor first numbs your throat with an anesthetic spray. You also may receive medicine to help you relax. The tube is passed through your mouth and esophagus to the stomach.

- **Biopsy:** The doctor uses an endoscope to remove tissue from the stomach. A pathologist checks the tissue under a microscope for cancer cells. A biopsy is the only sure way to know if cancer cells are present.

Staging

To plan the best treatment, your doctor needs to know the extent (stage) of the disease. The stage is based on whether the tumor has invaded nearby tissues, whether the cancer has spread, and if so, to what parts of the body. Stomach cancer can spread to the lymph nodes, liver, pancreas, and other organs. Sometimes staging is not complete until after surgery to remove the tumor and nearby lymph nodes.

Treatment

The choice of treatment depends mainly on the size and place of the tumor, the stage of disease, and your general health. Treatment for stomach cancer may involve surgery, chemotherapy, or radiation therapy. Many people have more than one type of treatment.

Surgery

Surgery is the most common treatment for stomach cancer. The type of surgery depends on the extent of the cancer. There are two main types of stomach cancer surgery:

- **Partial (Subtotal) Gastrectomy:** The surgeon removes the part of the stomach with cancer. The surgeon also may remove part of the esophagus or part of the small intestine. Nearby lymph nodes and other tissues may be removed.

- **Total Gastrectomy:** The doctor removes the entire stomach, nearby lymph nodes, parts of the esophagus and small intestine, and other tissues near the tumor. The spleen also may be removed. The surgeon then connects the esophagus directly to the small intestine. The surgeon makes a new "stomach" out of tissue from the intestine.

It is natural to be concerned about eating after surgery for stomach cancer. During surgery, the surgeon may place a feeding tube into your small intestine. This tube helps you get enough nutrition while you heal.

The time it takes to heal after surgery is different for each person. You may be uncomfortable for the first few days. Medicine can help control your pain. Before surgery, you should discuss the plan for pain relief with your doctor or nurse. After surgery, your doctor can adjust the plan if you need more pain relief.

Many people who have stomach surgery feel tired or weak for a while. The surgery also can cause constipation or diarrhea. These symptoms usually can be controlled with diet changes and medicine. Your health care team will watch for signs of bleeding, infection, or other problems that may require treatment.

Chemotherapy

Chemotherapy uses anticancer drugs to kill cancer cells. The drugs enter the bloodstream and can affect cancer cells all over the body.

Most people who receive chemotherapy have it after surgery. Radiation therapy may be given along with chemotherapy.

Anticancer drugs for stomach cancer are usually injected into a blood vessel. But some drugs may be given by mouth. You may have your treatment in a clinic at the hospital, at the doctor's office, or at home. Some people may need to stay in the hospital during treatment.

The side effects of chemotherapy depend mainly on the specific drugs and the dose. The drugs affect cancer cells and other cells that divide rapidly.

Radiation Therapy

Radiation therapy (also called radiotherapy) uses high-energy rays to kill cancer cells. It affects cells only in the treated area.

The radiation comes from a large machine outside the body. Most people go to a hospital or clinic for treatment. Treatments are usually five days a week for several weeks.

Side effects depend mainly on the dose of radiation and the part of your body that is treated. Radiation therapy to the abdomen may cause pain in the stomach or the intestine. You may have nausea and diarrhea. Also, your skin in the treated area may become red, dry, and tender.

♣ It's A Fact!!
Nutrition After Stomach Surgery

Weight loss after surgery for stomach cancer is common. You may need to change the types of food you eat. A registered dietitian can help you plan a diet that will give you the nutrition you need.

Another common problem after stomach surgery is dumping syndrome. This problem occurs when food or liquid enters the small intestine too fast. It can cause cramps, nausea, bloating, diarrhea, and dizziness. Eating smaller meals can help prevent dumping syndrome. Also, you may wish to cut down on very sweet foods and drinks, such as cookies, candy, soda, and juices. A registered dietitian can suggest foods to try. Also, your health care team may suggest medicine to control the symptoms.

You may need to take daily supplements of vitamins and minerals, such as calcium. You also may need injections of vitamin B12.

You are likely to become very tired during radiation therapy, especially in the later weeks of treatment. Resting is important, but doctors usually advise patients to try to stay as active as they can.

Although the side effects of radiation therapy can be distressing, your doctor can usually treat or control them. Also, side effects usually go away after treatment ends.

Follow-Up Care

Follow-up care after treatment for stomach cancer is important. Even when there are no longer any signs of cancer, the disease sometimes returns because undetected cancer cells remained somewhere in the body after treatment. Your doctor will monitor your recovery and check for recurrence of the cancer. Checkups help ensure that any changes in your health are noted and treated if needed. Checkups may include a physical exam, lab tests, x-rays, CT scans, endoscopy, or other tests. Between scheduled visits, you should contact the doctor if you have any health problems.

Part Four

Other Health Concerns Related To Tobacco Use

Chapter 33

Aneurysms

What Is An Aneurysm?

An aneurysm is a balloon-like bulge in an artery. Arteries are blood vessels that carry oxygen-rich blood from your heart to your body.

Arteries have thick walls to withstand normal blood pressure. However, certain medical problems, genetic conditions, and trauma can damage or injure artery walls. The force of blood pushing against the weakened or injured walls can cause an aneurysm.

An aneurysm can grow large and burst (rupture) or cause a dissection. Rupture causes dangerous bleeding inside the body. A dissection is a split in one or more layers of the artery wall. The split causes bleeding into and along the layers of the artery wall.

Both conditions are often fatal.

Overview

Most aneurysms occur in the aorta—the main artery that carries blood from the heart to the rest of the body. The aorta goes through the chest and abdomen.

About This Chapter: Text in the chapter is excerpted from "Aneurysm," National Heart Lung and Blood Institute, April 2009.

An aneurysm that occurs in the part of the aorta that's in the chest is called a thoracic aortic aneurysm. An aneurysm that occurs in the part of the aorta that's in the abdomen is called an abdominal aortic aneurysm.

Aneurysms also can occur in other arteries, but these types of aneurysm are less common. This chapter will focus on aortic aneurysms.

Outlook

When found in time, aortic aneurysms often can be successfully treated with medicines or surgery. Medicines may be given to lower blood pressure, relax blood vessels, and reduce the risk of rupture.

Large aortic aneurysms often can be repaired with surgery. During surgery, the weak or damaged portion of the aorta is replaced or reinforced.

Types Of Aneurysm

Aortic Aneurysms

The two types of aortic aneurysm are abdominal aortic aneurysm (AAA) and thoracic aortic aneurysm (TAA).

Abdominal Aortic Aneurysms

An aneurysm that occurs in the part of the aorta that's located in the abdomen is called an abdominal aortic aneurysm. AAAs account for three in four aortic aneurysms. They're found more often now than in the past because of computed tomography, or CT, scans done for other medical problems.

✤ It's A Fact!!

About 14,000 Americans die each year from aortic aneurysms. Most of the deaths result from rupture or dissection.

Early diagnosis and medical treatment can help prevent many cases of rupture and dissection. However, aneurysms can develop and become large before causing any symptoms. Thus, people who are at high risk for aneurysms can benefit from early, routine screening.

Small AAAs rarely rupture. However, an AAA can grow very large without causing symptoms. Thus, routine checkups and treatment for an AAA are important to prevent growth and rupture.

Thoracic Aortic Aneurysms

An aneurysm that occurs in the part of the aorta that's located in the chest and above the diaphragm is called a thoracic aortic aneurysm. TAAs account for one in four aortic aneurysms.

TAAs don't always cause symptoms, even when they're large. Only half of all people who have TAAs notice any symptoms. TAAs are found more often now than in the past because of chest CT scans done for other medical problems.

With a common type of TAA, the walls of the aorta weaken, and a section close to the heart enlarges. As a result, the valve between the heart and the aorta can't close properly. This allows blood to leak back into the heart.

A less common type of TAA can develop in the upper back, away from the heart. A TAA in this location may result from an injury to the chest, such as from a car crash.

Other Types Of Aneurysms

Brain Aneurysms

When an aneurysm occurs in an artery in the brain, it's called a cerebral aneurysm or brain aneurysm. Brain aneurysms also are sometimes called berry aneurysms because they're often the size of a small berry.

Most brain aneurysms cause no symptoms until they become large, begin to leak blood, or rupture. A ruptured brain aneurysm causes a stroke.

Peripheral Aneurysms

Aneurysms that occur in arteries other than the aorta and the brain arteries are called peripheral aneurysms. Common locations for peripheral aneurysms include the popliteal, femoral, and carotid arteries.

The popliteal arteries run down the back of the thighs, behind the knees. The femoral arteries are the main arteries in the groin. The carotid arteries are the two main arteries on each side of your neck.

Peripheral aneurysms aren't as likely to rupture or dissect as aortic aneurysms. However, blood clots can form in peripheral aneurysms. If a blood clot breaks away from the aneurysm, it can block blood flow through the artery.

If a peripheral aneurysm is large, it can press on a nearby nerve or vein and cause pain, numbness, or swelling.

What Causes An Aneurysm?

The force of blood pushing against the walls of an artery combined with damage or injury to the artery's walls can cause an aneurysm.

A number of factors can damage and weaken the walls of the aorta and cause aortic aneurysms.

- Aging, smoking, high blood pressure, and atherosclerosis are all factors that can damage or weaken the walls of the aorta. Atherosclerosis is the hardening and narrowing of the arteries due to the buildup of a fatty material called plaque.

- Rarely, infections, such as untreated syphilis (a sexually transmitted infection), can cause aortic aneurysms. Aortic aneurysms also can occur as a result of diseases that inflame the blood vessels, such as vasculitis.

- Family history also may play a role in causing aortic aneurysms.

In addition to the factors above, certain genetic conditions may cause thoracic aortic aneurysms (TAAs). Examples include Marfan syndrome, Loeys-Dietz syndrome, and Ehlers-Danlos syndrome (the vascular type).

These conditions can weaken the body's connective tissues and damage the aorta. People who have these conditions tend to develop aneurysms at a younger age and are at higher risk for rupture or dissection.

Trauma, such as a car accident, also can damage the aorta walls and lead to TAAs.

Researchers continue to look for other causes of aortic aneurysms. For example, they're looking for genetic mutations that may contribute to or cause aneurysms.

What Are The Signs And Symptoms Of An Aneurysm?

The signs and symptoms of an aortic aneurysm depend on the type of aneurysm, its location, and whether it has ruptured or is affecting other parts of the body.

Aneurysms can develop and grow for years without causing any signs or symptoms. They often don't cause signs or symptoms until they rupture, grow large enough to press on nearby parts of the body, or block blood flow.

Abdominal Aortic Aneurysms

Most abdominal aortic aneurysms (AAAs) develop slowly over years. They often don't have signs or symptoms unless they rupture. If you have an AAA, your doctor may feel a throbbing mass while checking your abdomen.

♣ It's A Fact!!

Certain factors put you at higher risk for an aortic aneurysm. These include the following:

- Male gender. Men are more likely than women to have abdominal aortic aneurysms (AAAs)—the most common type of aneurysm.

- Age. The risk for AAAs increases as you get older. These aneurysms are more likely to occur in people who are 65 or older.

- Smoking. Smoking can damage and weaken the walls of the aorta.

- Family history of aortic aneurysm. People who have family histories of aortic aneurysm are at higher risk of having one, and they may have aneurysms before the age of 65.

- Certain diseases and conditions that weaken the walls of the aorta.

- Car accidents or trauma also can injure the arteries and increase your risk for an aneurysm.

If you have any of these risk factors, talk with your doctor about whether you need to be screened for aneurysms.

When symptoms are present, they can include the following:

- A throbbing feeling in the abdomen
- Deep pain in your back or the side of your abdomen
- Steady, gnawing pain in your abdomen that lasts for hours or days

If an AAA ruptures, symptoms can include sudden, severe pain in your lower abdomen and back; nausea (feeling sick to your stomach) and vomiting; clammy, sweaty skin; lightheadedness; and a rapid heart rate when standing up.

Internal bleeding from a ruptured AAA can send you into shock. This is a life-threatening situation that requires emergency treatment.

Thoracic Aortic Aneurysms

A thoracic aortic aneurysm (TAA) may not cause symptoms until it dissects or grows large. Then, symptoms may include pain in your jaw, neck, back, or chest or coughing, hoarseness, or trouble breathing or swallowing.

A dissection is a split in one or more layers of the artery wall. The split causes bleeding into and along the layers of the artery wall.

If a TAA ruptures or dissects, you may feel sudden, severe pain starting in your upper back and moving down into your abdomen. You may have pain in your chest and arms, and you can quickly go into shock. Shock is a life-threatening condition in which the body's organs don't get enough blood flow.

✤ It's A Fact!!

A number of factors can damage and weaken the walls of the aorta and cause aortic aneurysms. Examples include aging, smoking, high blood pressure, atherosclerosis, infections, certain genetic conditions, and trauma. Family history also may play a role in causing aortic aneurysms.

The best way to prevent an aneurysm is to avoid the factors that put you at higher risk for one. You can't control all of the risk factors for aneurysm, but lifestyle changes can help you reduce your risks. Examples of lifestyle changes include following a healthy diet, doing physical activity, not smoking, and treating other medical conditions such as high blood pressure and high blood cholesterol.

How Is An Aneurysm Treated?

Aortic aneurysms are treated with medicines and surgery. A small aneurysm that's found early and isn't causing symptoms may not need treatment. Other aneurysms need to be treated.

The goals of treatment are to prevent the aneurysm from growing, prevent or reverse damage to other body structures, prevent or treat a rupture or dissection, and allow you to continue to do your normal daily activities.

Treatment for aortic aneurysms is based on the size of the aneurysm. Your doctor may recommend routine testing to make sure an aneurysm isn't getting bigger. This method usually is used for aneurysms that are smaller than five centimeters (about two inches) across.

How often you need testing (for example, every few months or every year) will be based on the size of the aneurysm and how fast it's growing. The larger it is and the faster it's growing, the more often you may need to be checked.

How Can An Aneurysm Be Prevented?

The best way to prevent an aortic aneurysm is to avoid the factors that put you at higher risk for one. You can't control all of the risk factors for aortic aneurysm, but lifestyle changes can help you reduce some risks.

Lifestyle changes include quitting smoking and controlling conditions such as high blood pressure and high blood cholesterol.

Talk to your doctor about programs and products that can help you quit smoking. Also try to avoid secondhand smoke.

Follow a healthy diet and be as physically active as you can. A healthy diet includes a variety of fruits, vegetables, and whole grains.

It also includes lean meats, poultry, fish, beans, and fat-free or low-fat milk or milk products. A healthy diet is low in saturated fat, trans fat, cholesterol, salt, and added sugar.

Follow your treatment plans for any other medical conditions you have. Take all of your medicines as prescribed.

Chapter 34

Asthma

Smoking And Asthma

You may have family photo albums full of people smoking at every type of event, from birthday parties to company picnics. That's because smoking was once accepted pretty much everywhere—even in doctor's offices. But that changed as we learned more about the health problems it causes.

If you have asthma, smoking is especially risky because of the damage it does to the lungs.

When someone smokes, he or she may cough, wheeze, and feel short of breath. This is because smoke irritates the airways, causing them to become swollen, narrow, and filled with sticky mucus. These are the same things that happen during an asthma flare-up. That's why smoking can cause asthma flare-ups to happen more often. Those flare-ups may be more severe and harder to control, even with medicine.

About This Chapter: Text in this chapter is from "Smoking and Asthma" June 2007, reprinted with permission from www.kidshealth.org. Copyright © 2007 The Nemours Foundation. This information was provided by KidsHealth, one of the largest resources online for medically reviewed health information written for parents, kids, and teens. For more articles like this one, visit www.KidsHealth.org, or www.TeensHealth.org.

If You Smoke

You may have started smoking because all your friends do or because you grew up in a house where lots of people smoked. Some people try smoking because they are curious or bored. No matter why you started, if you're thinking about quitting, it would probably help your asthma.

Smoking can undo the effect of any controller medicine you're taking. It also can force you to use your rescue medicine more often. It can also disturb your sleep by making you cough more at night and can affect how well you perform in sports or other physical activities. Worst of all, it can send you to the emergency department with a severe asthma flare-up.

> ✤ It's A Fact!!
> **The Smoking Habit**
>
> If you smoke, you aren't alone. Ninety percent of smokers start before they are 21. And many of them keep smoking because it is a highly addictive habit.
>
> Source: © 2007 Nemours Foundation.

If you decide to quit smoking, you don't have to go it alone. Seek the support of others who are also trying to quit. You also might ask your doctor about medication or different strategies that can help you crave cigarettes less.

If Other People Smoke

Even if you don't smoke, you may still run into smoky situations in restaurants, parties, or even at home if one of your family members smokes. Secondhand smoke is a known asthma trigger, so you'll want to avoid it as much as possible if you have asthma.

If you hang out with smokers or have a family member who smokes in the house, you are likely to have more frequent and severe asthma symptoms. You may have to take more medicine and your asthma may be harder to control. Finally, you may find yourself at the doctor's office or emergency department more often because of asthma symptoms.

There's not much you can do about other people's behavior, but you should let your friends and family know that what they are doing is making your asthma worse. Ask them not to smoke in your house or car. It's your air, after all.

✤ It's A Fact!!

- Less than 30% of people with asthma are taking all the essential actions recommended to reduce their exposure to indoor environmental asthma triggers.

- People with a written asthma management plan (AMP) are more likely to take actions to reduce exposure to environmental asthma triggers; however, only 30% of people with asthma have a written AMP.

- Almost three million children (11%) aged six and under, were reported to be exposed to environmental tobacco smoke (ETS) on a regular basis in their home. (Note: "regular" is defined as four or more days/week.)

- Major challenges remain in reducing ETS exposure for at-risk (sub-group) populations.

- ETS exposure is significantly higher in households at and below the poverty-level and in households with a lower educational level (less than a college degree).

- Parents account for the vast majority of exposure to ETS in homes.

- Children with asthma were just as likely to be exposed to ETS in their home as children in general.

Source: Excerpted from "Fact Sheet: National Survey on Environmental Management of Asthma and Children's Exposure to Environmental Tobacco Smoke," U.S. Environmental Protection Agency (www.epa.gov), 2004.

Chapter 35

Chronic Obstructive Pulmonary Disease (COPD)

What is COPD?

COPD, or chronic obstructive pulmonary disease, is a progressive disease that makes it hard to breathe. "Progressive" means the disease gets worse over time.

COPD can cause coughing that produces large amounts of mucus (a slimy substance), wheezing, shortness of breath, chest tightness, and other symptoms.

Cigarette smoking is the leading cause of COPD. Most people who have COPD smoke or used to smoke. Long-term exposure to other lung irritants, such as air pollution, chemical fumes, or dust, also may contribute to COPD.

To understand COPD, it helps to understand how the lungs work. The air that you breathe goes down your windpipe into tubes in your lungs called bronchial tubes, or airways.

The airways are shaped like an upside-down tree with many branches. At the end of the branches are tiny air sacs called alveoli.

The airways and air sacs are elastic. When you breathe in, each air sac fills up with air like a small balloon. When you breathe out, the air sac deflates and the air goes out.

About This Chapter: Text in this chapter is excerpted from "COPD," National Heart Lung and Blood Institute, March 2009.

In COPD, less air flows in and out of the airways because of one or more of the following:

- The airways and air sacs lose their elastic quality.
- The walls between many of the air sacs are destroyed.
- The walls of the airways become thick and inflamed (swollen).
- The airways make more mucus than usual, which tends to clog the airways.

In the United States, the term "COPD" includes two main conditions—emphysema and chronic obstructive bronchitis.

In emphysema, the walls between many of the air sacs are damaged, causing them to lose their shape and become floppy. This damage also can destroy the walls of the air sacs, leading to fewer and larger air sacs instead of many tiny ones.

In chronic obstructive bronchitis, the lining of the airways is constantly irritated and inflamed. This causes the lining to thicken. Lots of thick mucus forms in the airways, making it hard to breathe.

Most people who have COPD have both emphysema and chronic obstructive bronchitis. Thus, the general term "COPD" is more accurate.

✤ It's A Fact!! Outlook

COPD is a major cause of disability, and it's the fourth leading cause of death in the United States. More than 12 million people are currently diagnosed with COPD. An additional 12 million likely have the disease and don't even know it.

COPD develops slowly. Symptoms often worsen over time and can limit your ability to do routine activities. Severe COPD may prevent you from doing even basic activities like walking, cooking, or taking care of yourself.

Most of the time, COPD is diagnosed in middle-aged or older people. The disease isn't passed from person to person—you can't catch it from someone else.

COPD has no cure yet, and doctors don't know how to reverse the damage to the airways and lungs. However, treatments and lifestyle changes can help you feel better, stay more active, and slow the progress of the disease.

Source: National Heart Lung and Blood Institute, March 2009.

What causes COPD?

Most cases of COPD develop after long-term exposure to lung irritants that damage the lungs and the airways. In the United States, the most common irritant that causes COPD is cigarette smoke. Pipe, cigar, and other types of tobacco smoke also can cause COPD, especially if the smoke is inhaled. Secondhand smoke—that is, smoke in the air from other people smoking—also can irritate the lungs and contribute to COPD.

Breathing in air pollution and chemical fumes or dust from the environment or workplace also can contribute to COPD.

In rare cases, a genetic condition called alpha-1 antitrypsin deficiency may play a role in causing COPD. People who have this condition have low levels of alpha-1 antitrypsin (AAT)—a protein made in the liver.

Having a low level of the AAT protein can lead to lung damage and COPD if you're exposed to smoke or other lung irritants. If you have this condition and smoke, COPD can worsen very quickly.

Who is at risk for COPD?

The main risk factor for COPD is smoking. Most people who have COPD smoke or used to smoke. People who have a family history of COPD are more likely to get the disease if they smoke.

Long-term exposure to other lung irritants also is a risk factor for COPD. Examples of other lung irritants include air pollution and chemical fumes and dust from the environment or workplace.

Most people who have COPD are at least 40 years old when symptoms begin. Although it isn't common, people younger than 40 can have COPD. For example, this may happen if a person has alpha-1 antitrypsin deficiency, a genetic condition.

What are the signs and symptoms of COPD?

The signs and symptoms of COPD include the following:

- An ongoing cough or a cough that produces large amounts of mucus (often called "smoker's cough")

- Shortness of breath, especially with physical activity

- Wheezing (a whistling or squeaky sound when you breathe)

- Chest tightness

These symptoms often occur years before the flow of air into and out of the lungs declines. However, not everyone who has these symptoms has COPD. Likewise, not everyone who has COPD has these symptoms.

Some of the symptoms of COPD are similar to the symptoms of other diseases and conditions. Your doctor can determine if you have COPD.

COPD symptoms usually slowly worsen over time. At first, if symptoms are mild, you may not notice them, or you may adjust your lifestyle to make breathing easier. For example, you may take the elevator instead of the stairs.

♣ It's A Fact!!

Question: What about smoking as a cause of cough?

Answer: "Smoker's cough" is often due to a lung disease called chronic bronchitis, a disease most commonly caused by cigarette smoking. Irritation from the smoke causes increased mucus production and inflammation of the large air passages of the lungs. Most smokers do not seek medical attention for this cough, because they assume it is from smoking. Sometimes, however, a smoker is coughing from another cause. Just as in nonsmokers, the cough could be from upper airway cough syndrome (UACS), asthma, or gastroesophageal reflux disease (GERD), but it also could be a warning of an even more serious disorder, like lung cancer.

Question: If you are coughing from cigarette smoking and chronic bronchitis, will the cough go away if you stop smoking?

Answer: Typically, it will, but it can take 4 weeks to as long as a few months. If the cough seems different from your usual "smoker's cough," or if it persists despite stopping smoking for a month or longer, it definitely should be checked out by your doctor.

Source: Excerpted from "Information for Patients Complaining of Cough," reprinted with permission from The American College of Chest Physicians (www .chestnet.org), © 2009. All rights reserved.

♣ **It's A Fact!!**

If you have COPD, you may have frequent colds or flu. If your COPD is severe, you may have swelling in your ankles, feet, or legs; a bluish color on your lips due to low levels of oxygen in your blood; and shortness of breath.

Source: National Heart Lung and Blood Institute, March 2009.

Over time, symptoms may become bad enough to see a doctor. For example, you may get short of breath during physical exertion.

How severe your symptoms are depends on how much lung damage you have. If you keep smoking, the damage will occur faster than if you stop smoking. In severe COPD, you may have other symptoms, such as weight loss and lower muscle endurance.

Some severe symptoms may require treatment in a hospital. You—with the help of family members or friends, if you're unable—should seek emergency care if you experience these symptoms:

- You're having a hard time catching your breath or talking.

- Your lips or fingernails turn blue or gray. (This is a sign of a low oxygen level in your blood.)

- You're not mentally alert.

- Your heartbeat is very fast.

- The recommended treatment for symptoms that are getting worse isn't working.

How is COPD diagnosed?

Your doctor will diagnose COPD based on your signs and symptoms, your medical and family histories, and test results.

He or she may ask whether you smoke or have had contact with lung irritants, such as air pollution, chemical fumes, or dust. If you have an ongoing cough, your doctor may ask how long you've had it, how much you cough, and how much mucus comes up when you cough. He or she also may ask whether you have a family history of COPD.

Your doctor will examine you and use a stethoscope to listen for wheezing or other abnormal chest sounds.

You also may need one or more tests to diagnose COPD.

How is COPD treated?

COPD has no cure yet. However, treatments and lifestyle changes can help you feel better, stay more active, and slow the progress of the disease.

In addition to quitting smoking, other treatments for COPD may include medicines, vaccines, pulmonary rehabilitation (rehab), oxygen therapy, surgery, and managing complications.

- **Bronchodilators:** Bronchodilators relax the muscles around your airways. This helps open your airways and makes breathing easier. Most bronchodilators are taken using a device called an inhaler. This device allows the medicine to go right to your lungs.

♣ It's A Fact!!

Quitting smoking is the most important step you can take to treat COPD. Talk to your doctor about programs and products that can help you quit. Many hospitals have programs that help people quit smoking, or hospital staff can refer you to a program. Ask your family members and friends to support you in your efforts to quit. Also, try to avoid secondhand smoke.

Source: National Heart Lung and Blood Institute, March 2009.

- **Inhaled Glucocorticosteroids (Steroids):** Inhaled steroids are used for some people who have moderate or severe COPD. These medicines may reduce airway inflammation (swelling).

- **Vaccines:** The flu (influenza) can cause serious problems for people who have COPD. Flu shots can reduce your risk for the flu. The pneumococcal vaccine lowers your risk for pneumococcal pneumonia and its complications. People who have COPD are at higher risk for pneumonia than people who don't have COPD.

- **Pulmonary Rehabilitation:** Pulmonary rehab is a medically supervised program that helps improve the health and well-being of people who have lung problems. Rehab may include an exercise program, disease management training, and nutritional and psychological counseling. The program aims to help you stay more active and carry out your day-to-day activities.

- **Oxygen Therapy:** If you have severe COPD and low levels of oxygen in your blood, oxygen therapy can help you breathe better. For this treatment, you're given oxygen through nasal prongs or a mask. You may need extra oxygen all the time or just sometimes.

- **Surgery:** In rare cases, surgery may benefit some people who have COPD. Surgery usually is a last resort for people who have severe symptoms that have not improved from taking medicines. Surgeries for people who have COPD that is mainly related to emphysema include bullectomy (removal of one or more bullae—air spaces that form when the lung's air sacs are destroyed—from the lungs) and lung volume reduction surgery (LVRS, removed damaged tissues from the lungs). A lung transplant may be done for people who have very severe COPD.

- **Lung Transplant:** A lung transplant may benefit some people who have very severe COPD. During a lung transplant, your damaged lung is removed and replaced with a healthy lung from a deceased donor.

The goals of COPD treatment are to relieve your symptoms, slow the progress of the disease, improve your exercise tolerance (your ability to stay active), prevent and treat complications, and improve your overall health. To assist with your treatment, your family doctor may advise you to see a pulmonologist. This is a doctor who specializes in treating people who have lung problems.

COPD symptoms usually slowly worsen over time. However, they can become more severe suddenly. For instance, a cold, the flu, or a lung infection may cause your symptoms to quickly worsen. You may have a much harder time catching your breath. You also may have chest tightness, more coughing, changes in the color or amount of your sputum (spit), and a fever. Some severe symptoms may require treatment in a hospital.

How can COPD be prevented?

You can take steps to prevent COPD before it starts. If you already have COPD, you can take steps to prevent complications and slow the progress of the disease.

The best way to prevent COPD is to not start smoking or to quit smoking before you develop the disease. Smoking is the leading cause of COPD. If you smoke, talk to your doctor about programs and products that can help you quit. Many hospitals have programs that help people quit smoking, or hospital staff can refer you to a program. The National Heart, Lung, and Blood Institute's "Your Guide to a Healthy Heart" booklet has more information about how to quit smoking (visit www.nilbi.nih.gov for more information). Also, try to avoid secondhand smoke and other lung irritants that can contribute to COPD, such as air pollution, chemical fumes, and dust.

How can COPD progress and complications be slowed?

If you already have COPD, the most important step you can take is to quit smoking. This can help prevent complications and slow the progress of the disease. You also should avoid exposure to the lung irritants mentioned above.

Follow your treatments for COPD exactly as your doctor prescribes. They can help you breathe easier, stay more active, and avoid or manage severe symptoms.

Talk with your doctor about whether and when you should get flu and pneumonia vaccines. These vaccines can lower your chances of getting these illnesses, which are major health risks for people who have COPD.

How can a person with COPD manage to daily challenges?

COPD has no cure yet. However, you can take steps to manage your symptoms and slow the progress of the disease:

Avoid Lung Irritants: If you smoke, quit. Smoking is the leading cause of COPD. Talk to your doctor about programs and products that can help you quit. Many hospitals have programs that help people quit smoking, or hospital staff can refer you to a program.

Try to avoid secondhand smoke and other lung irritants that can contribute to COPD, such as air pollution, chemical fumes, and dust. Keep these irritants out of your home. If your home is painted or sprayed for insects, have it done when you can stay away for awhile.

Keep your windows closed and stay at home (if possible) when there's a lot of air pollution or dust outside.

Get Ongoing Care: If you have COPD, it's important to get ongoing medical care. Take all of your medicines as your doctor prescribes. Make sure to refill your prescriptions before they run out. Bring all of the medicines you're taking when you have medical checkups.

Talk with your doctor about whether and when you should get flu and pneumonia vaccines. Also, ask him or her about other diseases for which COPD may increase your risk, such as heart disease, lung cancer, and pneumonia.

Manage COPD And Its Symptoms: You can do things to help manage your disease and its symptoms. Depending on how severe your disease is, you may ask your family and friends for help with daily tasks. Do activities slowly. Put items that you need often in one place that's easy to reach.

Find very simple ways to cook, clean, and do other chores. Some people find it helpful to use a small table or cart with wheels to move things around and a pole or tongs with long handles to reach things. Ask for help moving things around in your house so that you will not need to climb stairs as often.

Keep your clothes loose, and wear clothes and shoes that are easy to put on and take off.

Prepare For Emergencies: If you have COPD, knowing when and where to seek help for your symptoms is important. You should seek emergency care if you have severe symptoms, such as trouble catching your breath or ta

Call your doctor if you notice that your symptoms are worsening or if you have signs of an infection, such as a fever. Your doctor may change or adjust your treatments to relieve and treat symptoms.

Keep phone numbers handy for your doctor, hospital, and someone who can take you for medical care. You also should have on hand directions to the doctor's office and hospital and a list of all the medicines you're taking.

Chapter 36

Deep Vein Thrombosis

What is deep vein thrombosis?

Deep vein thrombosis, or DVT, is a blood clot that forms in a vein deep in the body. Blood clots occur when blood thickens and clumps together.

Most deep vein blood clots occur in the lower leg or thigh. They also can occur in other parts of the body.

A blood clot in a deep vein can break off and travel through the bloodstream. The loose clot is called an embolus. When the clot travels to the lungs and blocks blood flow, the condition is called pulmonary embolism, or PE.

PE is a very serious condition. It can damage the lungs and other organs in the body and cause death.

Blood clots in the thigh are more likely to break off and cause PE than blood clots in the lower leg or other parts of the body.

Blood clots also can form in the veins closer to the skin's surface. However, these clots won't break off and cause PE.

What causes deep vein thrombosis?

Blood clots can form in your body's deep veins when damage occurs to a vein's inner lining. This damage may result from injuries caused by physical,

About This Chapter: Excerpted from "Deep Vein Thrombosis," National Heart Lung and Blood Institute, November 2007.

chemical, and biological factors. Such factors include surgery, serious injury, inflammation, or an immune response.

Blood clots can also form when blood flow is sluggish or slow. Lack of motion can cause sluggish or slowed blood flow. This may occur after surgery, if you're ill and in bed for a long time, or if you're traveling for a long time.

Another cause of blood clots is when your blood is thicker or more likely to clot than usual. Certain inherited conditions (such as factor V Leiden) increase blood's tendency to clot. This also is true of treatment with hormone replacement therapy or birth control pills.

Who is at risk for deep vein thrombosis?

Many factors increase your risk for deep vein thrombosis (DVT), including the following:

- A history of DVT.

- Disorders or factors that make your blood thicker or more likely to clot than normal. Certain inherited blood disorders (such as factor V Leiden) will do this. This also is true of treatment with hormone replacement therapy or using birth control pills.

- Injury to a deep vein from surgery, a broken bone, or other trauma.

- Slow blood flow in a deep vein from lack of movement. This may occur after surgery, if you're ill and in bed for a long time, or if you're traveling for a long time.

- Pregnancy and the first six weeks after giving birth.

- Recent or ongoing treatment for cancer.

- A central venous catheter. This is a tube placed in vein to allow easy access to the bloodstream for medical treatment.

- Being older than 60 (although DVT can occur in any age group).

- Being overweight or obese.

Your risk for DVT increases if you have more than one of the risk factors listed above.

✤ It's A Fact!!

The signs and symptoms of deep vein thrombosis (DVT) may be related to DVT itself or to pulmonary embolism (PE). See your doctor right away if you have symptoms of either. Both DVT and PE can cause serious, possibly life-threatening complications if not treated.

What are the signs and symptoms of DVT?

Only about half of the people with DVT have symptoms. These symptoms occur in the leg affected by the deep vein clot. They include the following:

- Swelling of the leg or along a vein in the leg
- Pain or tenderness in the leg, which you may feel only when standing or walking
- Increased warmth in the area of the leg that's swollen or in pain
- Red or discolored skin on the leg

Some people don't know they have DVT until they have signs or symptoms of PE. Symptoms of PE include:

- Unexplained shortness of breath
- Pain with deep breathing
- Coughing up blood

Rapid breathing and a fast heart rate also may be signs of PE.

How is deep vein thrombosis diagnosed?

Your doctor will diagnose deep vein thrombosis (DVT) based on your medical history, a physical exam, and the results from tests. He or she will identify your risk factors and rule out other causes for your symptoms.

To learn about your medical history, your doctor may ask about these things:

- Your overall health
- Any prescription medicines you're taking

- Any recent surgeries or injuries you've had

- Whether you've been treated for cancer

During the physical exam, your doctor will check your legs for signs of DVT. He or she also will check your blood pressure and your heart and lungs.

You may need one or more tests to find out whether you have DVT. The most common tests used to diagnose DVT are ultrasound (using sound waves to create pictures of blood flowing through the arteries and veins in the affected leg), a D-dimer test (measures a substance in the blood that's released when a blood clot dissolves), and venography (dye is injected into a vein, and then an x ray is taken of the leg). Other less common tests used to diagnose DVT include magnetic resonance imaging (MRI) and computed tomography (CT) scanning. These tests provide pictures of the inside of the body.

You may need blood tests to check whether you have an inherited blood clotting disorder that can cause DVT. You may have this type of disorder if you have repeated blood clots that can't be linked to another cause, or if you develop a blood clot in an unusual location, such as a vein in the liver, kidney, or brain.

If your doctor thinks that you have pulmonary embolism (PE), he or she may order extra tests, such as a ventilation perfusion scan (V/Q scan). The V/Q scan uses a radioactive material to show how well oxygen and blood are flowing to all areas of the lungs.

How can deep vein thrombosis be prevented?

If you're at risk for DVT or pulmonary embolism (PE), you can help prevent the condition by taking these steps:

- Seeing your doctor for regular checkups.

- Taking all medicines your doctor prescribes.

- Getting out of bed and moving around as soon as possible after surgery or illness. This lowers your chance of developing a blood clot.

- Exercising your lower leg muscles during long trips. This helps prevent a blood clot from forming.

If you've had DVT or PE before, you can help prevent future blood clots by following the above steps and by taking all medicines your doctor prescribes to prevent or treat blood clots, following up with your doctor for tests and treatment, and using compression stockings as your doctor directs to prevent swelling in your legs from DVT.

✔ Quick Tip

Your risk of developing deep vein thrombosis (DVT) while traveling is small. The risk increases if the travel time is longer than four hours or if you have other risk factors for DVT.

During long trips, it may help to take these precautions:

- Walk up and down the aisles of the bus, train, or airplane. If traveling by car, stop about every hour and walk around.

- Move your legs and flex and stretch your feet to encourage blood flow in your calves.

- Wear loose and comfortable clothing.

- Drink plenty of fluids and avoid alcohol.

- If you're at increased risk for DVT, your doctor may recommend wearing compression stockings during travel or taking a blood-thinning medicine before traveling.

How can a person with DVT manage to daily challenges?

If you've had a deep vein blood clot, you're at greater risk for another one. During treatment and after, it's important to check your legs for signs and symptoms of DVT. These include swollen areas, pain or tenderness, increased warmth in swollen or painful areas, or red or discolored skin on the legs. Contact your doctor right away if you have signs and symptoms of DVT.

Medicines that thin your blood and prevent blood clots are used to treat DVT. These medicines can thin your blood too much and cause bleeding (sometimes inside the body). This side effect can be life threatening. Bleeding may occur in the digestive system or the brain. Signs and symptoms of bleeding in the digestive system include bright red vomit or vomit that looks like coffee grounds, bright red blood in your stools or black, tarry stools, and pain in your abdomen. Signs and symptoms of bleeding in the brain include severe pain in your head, sudden changes in your vision, or sudden loss of movement in your arms or legs.

If you have any of these signs or symptoms, get treatment right away.

You also should seek treatment right away if you have a lot of bleeding after a fall or injury. This could be a sign that your DVT medicines have thinned your blood too much.

Talk to your doctor before taking any medicines other than your DVT medicines. This includes over-the-counter medicines. Aspirin, for example, also can thin your blood. Taking two medicines that thin your blood may raise your risk for bleeding.

Ask your doctor about how your diet affects these medicines. Foods that contain vitamin K can change how warfarin (a blood-thinning medicine used to treat DVT) works. Vitamin K is found in green, leafy vegetables and some oils, like canola and soybean oil. Your doctor can help you plan a balanced and healthy diet.

☞ Remember!!

You can take steps to prevent deep vein thrombosis (DVT). See your doctor regularly. Follow your treatment plan as your doctor prescribes, stay active if possible, and exercise your lower leg muscles during long trips. Contact your doctor at once if you have any symptoms of DVT or pulmonary embolism (PE).

Chapter 37

Digestive Disorders

Cigarette smoking causes many life-threatening diseases, including lung cancer, colon cancer, emphysema, and heart disease. Each year more than 400,000 Americans die from cigarette smoking. One in every five deaths in the United States is smoking related. Estimates show that about one-third of all adults smoke. Adult men seem to be smoking less, but women and teenagers of both sexes seem to be smoking more. Smoking affects the entire body, including the digestive system.

Harmful Effects Of Smoking On The Digestive System

Smoking can harm all parts of the digestive system, contributing to such common disorders as heartburn and peptic ulcers. Smoking increases the risk of Crohn disease, and possibly gallstones, which form when liquid stored in the gallbladder hardens into pieces of stone-like material. Smoking also damages the liver.

Heartburn

Heartburn is common with more than 50 million Americans having it at least once a month and about 15 million having it daily.

About This Chapter: From "Smoking and Your Digestive System," National Institute of Diabetes and Digestive and Kidney Diseases (www.niddk.nih.gov), February 2006.

Heartburn is a symptom of a syndrome called gastroesophageal reflux (GER). GER is when the natural acidic juices in the stomach flow backwards into the esophagus—the tube that connects the mouth to the stomach. Acidic juices are made by the stomach to help break down food. The stomach is naturally protected from acidic juices, but the esophagus does not have the same protection. Normally, a muscular valve at the lower end of the esophagus, called the lower esophageal sphincter (LES), keeps the acids in the stomach and out of the esophagus. Smoking, however, weakens the LES, which allows stomach acid to flow into the esophagus. When stomach acid comes in contact with the esophagus, the inner lining can become injured or damaged.

Peptic Ulcer

A peptic ulcer is a sore on the lining of the stomach or duodenum, which is the beginning of the small intestine. Peptic ulcers are common: One in ten Americans develops an ulcer at some time in his or her life. One cause of peptic ulcer is bacterial infection, but some ulcers are caused by long-term use of nonsteroidal anti-inflammatory agents, like aspirin and ibuprofen. In a few cases, cancerous tumors in the stomach or pancreas can cause ulcers. Peptic ulcers are not caused by stress or eating spicy food, but these can make ulcers worse.

Stomach acid also plays a part in producing ulcers. Normally, stomach acid is absorbed by the food we eat. The acid that is not absorbed by food enters the duodenum and is quickly neutralized by sodium bicarbonate, a salt-like substance made by the pancreas—an organ located next to the duodenum that aids in digestion. Some studies show that smoking reduces the amount of bicarbonate in the body, which causes problems in the neutralization of acid in the duodenum. Other studies suggest that cigarette smoking may increase the amount of acid secreted by the stomach over time.

Liver Disease

The liver is an important organ that has many tasks. The liver is responsible for processing drugs, alcohol, and other toxins and removing them from the body. Research shows that smoking harms the liver's ability to process such substances. In some cases, if the liver has been damaged from cigarette smoking, the dose of medication necessary to treat an illness may be affected. Research also suggests that smoking can worsen liver disease caused by drinking too much alcohol.

❖ It's A Fact!!

Research has shown that people who smoke cigarettes are more likely to develop an ulcer. If people with an ulcer keep smoking, their ulcer may not heal; or it may take longer than usual to heal. People have a better chance of their ulcer healing if they stop smoking compared to treating their ulcer with medication while still smoking. Smoking also increases people's risk of infection from a bacterium called Helicobacter pylori and increases the risk of ulceration from alcohol and over-the-counter pain relievers.

Crohn Disease

Crohn disease causes swelling deep in the lining of the intestine. The disease, which causes pain and diarrhea, most often affects the small intestine, but it can occur anywhere in the digestive tract. Research shows that current and former smokers have a higher risk of developing Crohn disease than nonsmokers. Among people with Crohn disease, smoking is linked with a higher rate of relapse, repeat surgery, and the need for drug therapy. Women have a higher risk of relapsing and needing surgery and treatment than men whether they are current or former smokers. Why smoking increases the risk of Crohn's disease is unknown, but some researchers believe that smoking might lower the intestines defenses, decrease blood flow to the intestines, or cause immune system changes that result in inflammation.

Gallstones

Several studies show that smoking may increase the risk of developing gallstones and that the risk may be higher for women. However, research results on this topic are not consistent and more study is needed.

Reversing Smoking-Related Damage

Some of the effects of smoking on the digestive system appear to be of short duration. For example, the effect of smoking on the pancreas's bicarbonate production does not appear to last. Within a half-hour after smoking, the production of bicarbonate returns to normal. The effects of smoking on how the liver handles drugs also disappear when a person stops smoking. However, people who no longer smoke still remain at risk for Crohn disease.

Chapter 38

Eye Disease

Smoking is as bad for your eyes as it is for the rest of your body. Research has linked smoking to an increased risk of developing age-related macular degeneration, cataract, and optic nerve damage, all of which can lead to blindness.

Cataract

What is a cataract?

A cataract is a clouding of the lens in the eye that affects vision. Most cataracts are related to aging. Cataracts are very common in older people. By age 80, more than half of all Americans either have a cataract or have had cataract surgery.

A cataract can occur in either or both eyes. It cannot spread from one eye to the other.

Although most cataracts are related to aging, there are other types of cataract:

- **Secondary Cataract:** Cataracts can form after surgery for other eye problems, such as glaucoma. Cataracts also can develop in people who have other health problems, such as diabetes. Cataracts are sometimes linked to steroid use.

About This Chapter: Text in this chapter is excerpted from "Eye Health Tips," National Eye Institute (NEI), "Facts about Cataract," NEI, and "Facts about Age-Related Macular Degeneration," NEI, February 2010.

- **Traumatic cataract:** Cataracts can develop after an eye injury, sometimes years later.

- **Congenital cataract:** Some babies are born with cataracts or develop them in childhood, often in both eyes. These cataracts may be so small that they do not affect vision. If they do, the lenses may need to be removed.

- **Radiation cataract:** Cataracts can develop after exposure to some types of radiation.

What causes cataracts?

The lens lies behind the iris and the pupil. It works much like a camera lens. It focuses light onto the retina at the back of the eye, where an image is recorded. The lens also adjusts the eye's focus, letting us see things clearly both up close and far away. The lens is made of mostly water and protein. The protein is arranged in a precise way that keeps the lens clear and lets light pass through it.

But as we age, some of the protein may clump together and start to cloud a small area of the lens. This is a cataract. Over time, the cataract may grow larger and cloud more of the lens, making it harder to see.

Researchers suspect that there are several causes of cataract, such as smoking and diabetes. Or, it may be that the protein in the lens just changes from the wear and tear it takes over the years.

How can cataracts affect my vision?

Age-related cataracts can affect your vision in two ways:

- Clumps of protein reduce the sharpness of the image reaching the retina. The lens consists mostly of water and protein. When the protein clumps up, it clouds the lens and reduces the light that reaches the retina. The clouding may become severe enough to cause blurred vision. Most age-related cataracts develop from protein clumpings.

- The clear lens slowly changes to a yellowish/brownish color, adding a brownish tint to vision. As the clear lens slowly colors with age, your vision gradually may acquire a brownish shade. At first, the amount of tinting may be small and may not cause a vision problem. Over time, increased tinting may make it more difficult to read and perform other routine activities. This gradual change in the amount of tinting does not affect the sharpness of the image transmitted to the retina. If you have advanced lens discoloration, you may not be able to identify blues and purples. You may be wearing what you believe to be a pair of black socks, only to find out from friends that you are wearing purple socks.

When are you most likely to have a cataract?

The term "age-related" is a little misleading. You don't have to be a senior citizen to get this type of cataract. In fact, people can have an age-related cataract in their 40s and 50s. But during middle age, most cataracts are small and do not affect vision. It is after age 60 that most cataracts steal vision.

Who is at risk for cataract?

The risk of cataract increases as you get older. Other risk factors for cataract include the following:

- Certain diseases such as diabetes
- Personal behavior such as smoking and alcohol use
- The environment such as prolonged exposure to sunlight

What can I do to protect my vision?

Wearing sunglasses and a hat with a brim to block ultraviolet sunlight may help to delay cataract. If you smoke, stop. Researchers also believe good nutrition can help reduce the risk of age-related cataract. They recommend eating green leafy vegetables, fruit, and other foods with antioxidants.

Age-Related Macular Degeneration

What is age-related macular degeneration?

Age-related macular degeneration (AMD) is a disease associated with aging that gradually destroys sharp, central vision. Central vision is needed for seeing objects clearly and for common daily tasks such as reading and driving. AMD causes no pain.

✎ **What's It Mean?**

Lens: The lens is a clear part of the eye that helps to focus light, or an image, on the retina.

Macula: The macula, located in the center of the retina, is the part of the eye that allows you to see fine detail.

Retina: The retina is the light-sensitive tissue at the back of the eye. It instantly converts light, or an image, into electrical impulses and then sends these impulses, or nerve signals, to the brain.

Source: National Eye Institute, February 2010.

In some cases, AMD advances so slowly that people notice little change in their vision. In others, the disease progresses faster and may lead to a loss of vision in both eyes. AMD is a leading cause of vision loss in Americans 60 years of age and older.

Where is the macula?

The macula is located in the center of the retina, the light-sensitive tissue at the back of the eye. The retina instantly converts light, or an image, into electrical impulses. The retina then sends these impulses, or nerve signals, to the brain.

What are wet and dry AMD?

Wet AMD occurs when abnormal blood vessels behind the retina start to grow under the macula. These new blood vessels tend to be very fragile and often leak blood and fluid. The blood and fluid raise the macula from its normal place at the back of the eye. Damage to the macula occurs rapidly.

With wet AMD, loss of central vision can occur quickly. Wet AMD is also known as advanced AMD. It does not have stages like dry AMD.

An early symptom of wet AMD is that straight lines appear wavy. If you notice this condition or other changes to your vision, contact your eye care professional at once. You need a comprehensive dilated eye exam.

Dry AMD occurs when the light-sensitive cells in the macula slowly break down, gradually blurring central vision in the affected eye. As dry AMD gets worse, you may see a blurred spot in the center of your vision. Over time, as less of the macula functions, central vision is gradually lost in the affected eye.

The most common symptom of dry AMD is slightly blurred vision. You may have difficulty recognizing faces. You may need more light for reading and other tasks. Dry AMD generally affects both eyes, but vision can be lost in one eye while the other eye seems unaffected.

One of the most common early signs of dry AMD is drusen.

What are drusen?

Drusen are yellow deposits under the retina. They often are found in people over age 60. Your eye care professional can detect drusen during a comprehensive dilated eye exam.

Drusen alone do not usually cause vision loss. In fact, scientists are unclear about the connection between drusen and AMD. They do know that an increase in the size or number of drusen raises a person's risk of developing either advanced dry AMD or wet AMD. These changes can cause serious vision loss.

✤ It's A Fact!!

The following age-related conditions are thought to occur at higher rates in smokers than nonsmokers:

- **Cataracts:** Quitting smoking reduces your chances of needing cataract surgery in the future, although not to the level seen with nonsmokers.

- **Age-Related Macular Degeneration (AMD):** AMD is a leading cause of blindness in older people. Symptoms of macular degeneration include a loss of central vision, which makes it difficult to read.

Source: Excerpted from "Smoking," © 2010 A.D.A.M, Inc. Reprinted with permission.

Who is at risk for AMD?

The greatest risk factor is age. Although AMD may occur during middle age, studies show that people over age 60 are clearly at greater risk than other age groups. For instance, a large study found that people in middle-age have about a two percent risk of getting AMD, but this risk increased to nearly 30% in those over age 75.

Other risk factors include the following:

- **Smoking:** Smoking may increase the risk of AMD.
- **Obesity:** Research studies suggest a link between obesity and the progression of early and intermediate stage AMD to advanced AMD.
- **Race:** Whites are much more likely to lose vision from AMD than African Americans.
- **Family History:** Those with immediate family members who have AMD are at a higher risk of developing the disease.
- **Gender:** Women appear to be at greater risk than men.

Can lifestyle make a difference?

Your lifestyle can play a role in reducing your risk of developing AMD.

- Eat a healthy diet high in green leafy vegetables and fish.
- Don't smoke.
- Maintain normal blood pressure.
- Watch your weight.
- Exercise.

Chapter 39

Heart Attacks

Understanding Heart Attacks

A heart attack occurs when blood flow to a section of heart muscle becomes blocked. If the flow of blood isn't restored quickly, the section of heart muscle becomes damaged from lack of oxygen and begins to die.

Heart attack is a leading killer of both men and women in the United States. But fortunately, today there are excellent treatments for heart attack that can save lives and prevent disabilities.

Get Help Quickly

Acting fast at the first sign of heart attack symptoms can save your life and limit damage to your heart. Treatment is most effective when started within one hour of the beginning of symptoms.

The most common heart attack signs and symptoms are the following:

• Chest discomfort or pain—uncomfortable pressure, squeezing, fullness, or pain in the center of the chest that can be mild or strong. This discomfort or pain lasts more than a few minutes or goes away and comes back.

About This Chapter: Text in this chapter is from "Heart Attacks," National Heart Lung and Blood Institute, March 2008.

- Upper body discomfort in one or both arms, the back, neck, jaw, or stomach.

- Shortness of breath may occur with or before chest discomfort.

- Other signs include nausea (feeling sick to your stomach), vomiting, lightheadedness or fainting, or breaking out in a cold sweat.

If you think you or someone you know may be having a heart attack:

> ✎ **What's It Mean?**
>
> Treatment for heart attacks is most effective when started within one hour of the beginning of symptoms. If you think you or someone you're with is having a heart attack, call 911 right away.
>
> Source: National Heart Lung and Blood Institute, March 2008.

- Call 911 within a few minutes—five at the most—of the start of symptoms.

- If your symptoms stop completely in less than five minutes, still call your doctor.

- Only take an ambulance to the hospital. Going in a private car can delay treatment.

- Take a nitroglycerin pill if your doctor has prescribed this type of medicine.

Outlook

Each year, about 1.1 million people in the United States have heart attacks, and almost half of them die. CAD, which often results in a heart attack, is the leading killer of both men and women in the United States.

Many more people could recover from heart attacks if they got help faster. Of the people who die from heart attacks, about half die within an hour of the first symptoms and before they reach the hospital.

Other Names For A Heart Attack

- Myocardial infarction or MI

- Acute myocardial infarction or AMI

- Acute coronary syndrome

- Coronary thrombosis

- Coronary occlusion

Heart Attack Causes

Most heart attacks occur as a result of coronary artery disease (CAD). CAD is the buildup over time of a material called plaque on the inner walls of the coronary arteries. Eventually, a section of plaque can break open, causing a blood clot to form at the site. A heart attack occurs if the clot becomes large enough to cut off most or all of the blood flow through the artery.

> ♣ **It's A Fact!!**
>
> All forms of tobacco raise the risk of heart attacks. Smoking, chewing tobacco, and being exposed to second-hand smoke greatly increase the risk of a heart attack. In some cases, the risk of heart problems in people who smoke or are exposed to smoke may be three times greater. The risk of a heart attack among those who stopped smoking may slowly decrease over time.
>
> Source: Excerpted from "Smoking," © 2010 A.D.A.M, Inc. Reprinted with permission.

The blocked blood flow prevents oxygen-rich blood from reaching the part of the heart muscle fed by the artery. The lack of oxygen damages the heart muscle. If the blockage isn't treated quickly, the damaged heart muscle begins to die.

Heart attack also can occur due to problems with the very small, microscopic blood vessels of the heart. This condition is called microvascular disease. It's believed to be more common in women than in men.

Another less common cause of heart attack is a severe spasm (tightening) of a coronary artery that cuts off blood flow through the artery. These spasms can occur in coronary arteries that don't have CAD. It's not always clear what causes a coronary artery spasm, but sometimes it can be related to the following:

- Taking certain drugs, such as cocaine

- Emotional stress or pain

- Exposure to extreme cold

- Cigarette smoking

Heart Attack Risk Factors

Certain risk factors make it more likely that you will develop coronary artery disease (CAD) and have a heart attack. Some risk factors for heart attack can be controlled, while others can't.

Major risk factors for heart attack that you can control include the following:

- Smoking

- High blood pressure

- High blood cholesterol

- Overweight and obesity

- Physical inactivity

- Diabetes (high blood sugar)

Risk factors that you can't change include age, family history, and other conditions:

- **Age:** Risk increases for men older than 45 years and for women older than 55 years (or after menopause).

- **Family History Of Early CAD:** Your risk increases if your father or a brother was diagnosed with CAD before 55 years of age, or if your mother or a sister was diagnosed with CAD before 65 years of age.

- **Related Conditions:** Certain CAD risk factors tend to occur together. When they do, it's called metabolic syndrome. In general, a person with metabolic syndrome is twice as likely to develop heart disease and five times as likely to develop diabetes as someone without metabolic syndrome.

Signs And Symptoms Of A Heart Attack

Not all heart attacks begin with a sudden, crushing pain that is often shown on TV or in the movies. The warning signs and symptoms of a heart attack aren't the same for everyone. Many heart attacks start slowly as mild pain or discomfort. Some people don't have symptoms at all (this is called a silent heart attack).

Chest Pain Or Discomfort

The most common symptom of heart attack is chest pain or discomfort. Most heart attacks involve discomfort in the center of the chest that lasts for more than a few minutes or goes away and comes back. The discomfort can feel like uncomfortable pressure, squeezing, fullness, or pain. It can be mild or severe. Heart attack pain can sometimes feel like indigestion or heartburn.

The symptoms of angina can be similar to the symptoms of a heart attack. Angina is pain in the chest that occurs in people with coronary artery disease, usually when they're active. Angina pain usually lasts for only a few minutes and goes away with rest. Angina that doesn't go away or that changes from its usual pattern (occurs more frequently or occurs at rest) can be a sign of the beginning of a heart attack and should be checked by a doctor right away.

Other Common Signs And Symptoms

There are other common signs and symptoms that a person can have during a heart attack:

- Upper body discomfort in one or both arms, the back, neck, jaw, or stomach
- Shortness of breath may often occur with or before chest discomfort
- Nausea (feeling sick to your stomach), vomiting, lightheadedness or fainting, or breaking out in a cold sweat

Not everyone having a heart attack experiences the typical symptoms. If you've already had a heart attack, your symptoms may not be the same for another one. The more signs and symptoms you have, the more likely it is that you're having a heart attack.

Act Fast

Sometimes the signs and symptoms of a heart attack happen suddenly, but they can also develop slowly, over hours, days, and even weeks before a heart attack occurs.

Know the warning signs of a heart attack so you can act fast to get treatment for yourself or someone else. The sooner you get emergency help, the less damage there will be to your heart.

Call 911 for help within five minutes if you think you may be having a heart attack or if your chest pain doesn't go away as it usually does when you take prescribed medicine.

Don't drive yourself or anyone else to the hospital. Call an ambulance so that medical personnel can begin life-saving treatment on the way to the emergency room.

Diagnosing A Heart Attack

The diagnosis of heart attack is based on your symptoms, your personal and family medical history, and the results of diagnostic tests.

EKG (Electrocardiogram)

This test detects and records the electrical activity of the heart. Certain changes in the appearance of the electrical waves on an EKG are strong evidence of a heart attack. An EKG also can show if you're having arrhythmias (abnormal heartbeats), which a heart attack (and other conditions) can cause.

Blood Tests

During a heart attack, heart muscle cells die and burst open, letting certain proteins out in the bloodstream. Blood tests can measure the amount of these proteins in the bloodstream. Higher than normal levels of these proteins in the bloodstream is evidence of a heart attack.

Commonly used blood tests include troponin tests, CK or CK–MB tests, and serum myoglobin tests. Blood tests are often repeated to check for changes over time.

Coronary Angiography

Coronary angiography is a special x-ray exam of the heart and blood vessels. It's often done during a heart attack to help pinpoint blockages in the coronary arteries.

The doctor passes a catheter (a thin, flexible tube) through an artery in your arm or groin (upper thigh) and threads it to your heart. This procedure—called cardiac catheterization—is part of coronary angiography.

A dye that can be seen on x ray is injected into the bloodstream through the tip of the catheter. The dye lets the doctor study the flow of blood through the heart and blood vessels.

If a blockage is found, another procedure, called angioplasty, may be used to restore blood flow through the artery. Sometimes during angioplasty, the doctor will place a stent (a small mesh tube) in the artery to help keep the artery open.

Prevented Heart Attacks

Lowering your risk factors for coronary artery disease (CAD) can help you prevent a heart attack. Even if you already have CAD, you can still take steps to lower your risk of heart attack.

Reducing the risk of heart attack usually means making healthy lifestyle choices. You also may need treatment for medical conditions that raise your risk.

Healthy Lifestyle Choices

Healthy lifestyle choices to help prevent heart attack:

- Follow a low-fat diet rich in fruits and vegetables. Pay careful attention to the amounts and types of fat in your diet. Lower your salt intake. These changes can help lower high blood pressure and high blood cholesterol.

- Lose weight if you're overweight or obese.

- Quit smoking.

- Participate in physical activity to improve heart fitness. Ask your doctor how much and what kinds of physical activity are safe for you.

Treat Related Conditions

In addition to making lifestyle changes, you can help prevent heart attacks by treating conditions you have that make a heart attack more likely:

- **High Blood Cholesterol:** You may need medicine to lower your cholesterol if diet and exercise aren't enough.

- **High Blood Pressure:** You may need medicine to keep your blood pressure under control.

- **Diabetes (High Blood Sugar):** If you have diabetes, control your blood sugar levels through diet and physical activity (as your doctor recommends). If needed, take medicine as prescribed.

Have An Emergency Action Plan

Make sure that you have an emergency action plan in case you or someone else in your family has a heart attack. This is especially important if you're at high risk or have already had a heart attack.

Talk with your doctor about the signs and symptoms of heart attack, when you should call 911, and steps you can take while waiting for medical help to arrive.

Life After A Heart Attack

Many people survive heart attacks and live active and full lives. If you get help quickly, treatment can limit the damage to your heart muscle. Less heart damage improves your chances for a better quality of life after a heart attack.

Medical Follow-up

After a heart attack, you will need treatment for coronary artery disease to prevent another heart attack. Your doctor may recommend lifestyle changes, such as quitting smoking, following a healthy diet, increasing your physical activity, and losing weight, if needed. Your doctor may prescribe medicines to control chest pain or discomfort, blood pressure, blood cholesterol, and your heart's workload. Your doctor may also suggest that you participate in a cardiac rehabilitation program.

Returning To Normal Activities

After a heart attack, most people without chest pain or discomfort or other complications can safely return to most of their normal activities within a few weeks. Most can begin walking immediately. Sexual activity also can begin within a few weeks for most patients. Discuss with your doctor a safe schedule for returning to your normal activities.

If allowed by state law, driving can usually begin within a week for most patients who don't have chest pain or discomfort or other complications. Each state has rules about driving a motor vehicle following a serious illness. People with complications shouldn't drive until their symptoms have been stable for a few weeks.

Anxiety And Depression After A Heart Attack

After a heart attack, many people worry about having another heart attack. Sometimes they feel depressed and have trouble adjusting to the new lifestyle that's needed to limit further heart trouble. Your doctor may recommend medicine or professional counseling if you have depression or anxiety. Physical activity can improve mental well-being, but you should consult with your doctor before starting any fitness activities.

☞ Remember!!

- A heart attack occurs when blood flow to a section of heart muscle becomes blocked. If the flow of blood isn't restored quickly, the section of heart muscle becomes damaged from lack of oxygen and begins to die.

- Heart attack is a leading killer of both men and women in the United States.

- Today there are excellent treatments for heart attack that can save lives and prevent disabilities.

- Treatment is most effective when started within one hour of the beginning of symptoms.

- Unfortunately, many heart attack victims wait two hours or more after their symptoms begin before they seek medical help. This delay can result in lasting heart damage or death.

- If you think you or someone with you is having a heart attack, call 911 right away.

- Heart attacks occur most often as a result of a condition called coronary artery disease (CAD).

- Heart attack also can be caused by a condition called microvascular disease, which involves the microscopic blood vessels of the heart. Less commonly, a spasm (tightening) of a coronary artery can cause a heart attack.

- Certain risk factors increase the changes of developing CAD and having a heart attack (for example, age, a family history of CAD, smoking, and being overweight or obese). Some risk factors can't be controlled, while others can.

Source: National Heart Lung and Blood Institute, March 2008.

Risk Of A Repeat Heart Attack

Once you've had a heart attack, you're at higher risk for another one. It's important to know the difference between angina and a heart attack. The pain of angina usually occurs after exertion and goes away in a few minutes when you rest or take medicine as directed. During a heart attack, the pain is usually more severe than angina, and it doesn't go away when you rest or take medicine. If you don't know whether your chest pain is angina or a heart attack, call 911.

Remember, the symptoms of a second heart attack may not be the same as those of a first heart attack. Don't take a chance if you're in doubt. Always call 911 within five minutes if you or someone you're with has symptoms of a heart attack.

Unfortunately, most heart attack victims wait two hours or more after their symptoms begin before they seek medical help. This delay can result in lasting heart damage or death.

Chapter 40

Musculoskeletal Disorders

Impact Of Smoking On Health

Smoking remains the number one cause of preventable death. Each year more than 400,000 people in the United States alone die from tobacco-related diseases. In fact, smokers can expect to live seven to ten years less than nonsmokers.

Smoking is linked to heart and respiratory diseases and to several cancers. In addition, smoking has a significant impact on your bones and joints.

Effects Of Smoking On Musculoskeletal Health

Every tissue in the human body is affected by smoking, but many effects are reversible. By avoiding or quitting smoking, you can reduce your risk for incurring many conditions. Quitting smoking can also help your body regain some of its normal healthy functioning.

Here's what scientists have found about the relationship between smoking and musculoskeletal health.

- Smoking increases your risk of developing osteoporosis.

About This Chapter: Text in this chapter is from "Smoking and Musculoskeletal Health," reproduced with permission from *Your Orthopaedic Connection*. Rosemont, IL, American Academy of Orthopaedic Surgeons, © 2009.

- Smoking has a detrimental effect on bone density.

- Studies have shown that smoking reduces the blood supply to bones and that nicotine slows the production of bone-forming cells (osteoblasts) and impairs the absorption of calcium. With less bone mineral, smokers develop fragile bones (osteoporosis).

- Smoking also reduces the protective effect of estrogen replacement therapy.

- Smoking increases your risk of a hip fracture as you age.

- Osteoporosis is often a risk factor in hip fractures. Elderly smokers have a 41% increase in the rate of hip fracture.

♣ It's A Fact!!

Smoking has many harmful effects on bones and joints:

- Smoking can slow the process that adds calcium to bones, making them stronger. Women who smoke are at high risk for loss of bone density and osteoporosis.

- Postmenopausal women who smoke have a significantly greater risk for hip fracture than those who do not.

- Men who smoke may have more severe symptoms of knee arthritis, according to a study published in the Annals of Rheumatic Disease.

- Smokers are more apt to develop degenerative disorders and injuries in the spine.

- Smokers have more trouble recovering from surgeries.

- Smokers whose jobs involve lifting heavy objects are more likely to develop low back pain than nonsmokers.

Source: "Smoking," © 2010 A.D.A.M, Inc. Reprinted with permission.

Smoking increases your risk of developing exercise-related injuries.

- Rotator cuff (shoulder) tears in smokers are nearly twice as large as those in nonsmokers.

- Additionally, a study of young Army recruits showed that smokers were 1.5 times more likely to suffer overuse injuries such as bursitis or tendonitis than nonsmokers.

- Smokers were also more likely to suffer traumatic injuries, such as sprains or fractures.

Smoking has a detrimental effect on fracture and wound healing.

- Fractures take longer to heal in smokers because of the harmful effects of nicotine on the production of bone-forming cells.

- Smokers also have a higher rate of complications after surgery than nonsmokers, and outcomes are less satisfactory.

- Smoking has a detrimental effect on athletic performance.

- Because smoking slows lung growth and impairs lung function, there is less oxygen available for muscles used in sports. Smokers suffer from shortness of breath almost three times more often than nonsmokers. Smokers cannot run or walk as fast or as far as nonsmokers.

- Smoking is associated with low back pain and rheumatoid arthritis.

Chapter 41

Nicotine Poisoning

Nicotine is a bitter-tasting compound that naturally occurs in large amounts in the leaves of tobacco plants.

Nicotine poisoning results from too much nicotine. Acute nicotine poisoning usually occurs in young children who accidentally chew on nicotine gum or patches.

This is for information only and not for use in the treatment or management of an actual poison exposure. If you have an exposure, you should call your local emergency number (such as 911) or the National Poison Control Center at 800-222-1222.

Poisonous Ingredient

- Nicotine

Where Found

- Chewing tobacco
- Nicotine gum (Nicorette)
- Pipe tobacco
- Tobacco leaves

- Cigarettes
- Nicotine patches (Habitrol, Nicoderm)
- Some insecticides

Note: This list may not be all-inclusive.

Symptoms

- Abdominal cramps

- Agitation, restlessness, or excitement

- Muscular twitching

- Breathing—rapid

- Breathing—stops

- Burning sensation in mouth

- Coma

- Confusion

- Convulsions

- Depression

- Difficulty breathing

- Drooling (increased salivation)

- Fainting

- Headache

- Heartbeat—pounding and rapid, followed by slow heart rate

- High blood pressure, which then drops

- Vomiting

- Weakness

> ✤ **It's A Fact!!**
> ## Outlook (Prognosis)
>
> How well a patient does depends on the amount of poison swallowed and how quickly treatment was received. The faster a patient gets medical help, the better the chance for recovery.
>
> A nicotine overdose may cause seizures or death. However, unless there are complications, long-term effects from nicotine are uncommon.

Home Care

Seek immediate medical help. Do not make a person throw up unless told to do so by Poison Control or a health care professional. If the chemical is on the skin, wash with soap and lots of water for at least 15 minutes.

Before Calling Emergency

Determine the following information:

- The patient's age, weight, and condition

- Name of product (as well as the ingredients and strength if known)

- When it was swallowed or inhaled

- The amount swallowed or inhaled

However, do not delay calling for help if this information is not immediately available.

Poison Control

The National Poison Control Center (800-222-1222) can be called from anywhere in the United States. This national hotline number will let you talk to experts in poisoning. They will give you further instructions.

This is a free and confidential service. All local poison control centers in the United States use this national number. You should call if you have any questions about poisoning or poison prevention. It does not need to be an emergency. You can call for any reason, 24 hours a day, seven days a week.

What To Expect At The Emergency Room

The health care provider will measure and monitor the patient's vital signs, including temperature, pulse, breathing rate, and blood pressure. Symptoms will be treated as appropriate. The patient may receive:

- Activated charcoal

- Tube through the mouth or nose into the stomach to wash out the stomach (gastric lavage)

Chapter 42

Periodontal Disease

Want Some Life Saving Advice? Ask Your Dental Hygienist About Tobacco Use And Periodontal Disease

As if the oral effects of bad breath, stained teeth, loss of taste and smell, mouth (canker) sores, failure of dental implants, and oral cancer weren't enough, tobacco use is implicated in the gum recession, bone loss, and tooth loss associated with periodontal (gum) disease.

Smokers who smoked less than a half a pack of cigarettes per day are almost three times more likely than nonsmokers to have periodontitis, according to a study by researchers at the Centers for Disease Control and Prevention in Atlanta, Georgia. The same study found that those who smoked more than a pack and a half of cigarettes per day had almost six times the risk.

Periodontal diseases, including gingivitis and periodontitis, are severe infections, and if left untreated, they can lead to tooth loss. Periodontal disease is a chronic bacterial infection that affects the gum tissue, bone, and attachment fibers that support the teeth and hold them in place in the jaw bone. It occurs when plaque (a soft, sticky, colorless film of bacteria) forms on the teeth and at the gumline and infects the gum tissue, causing gingivitis (inflammation and reddening of the gums). If periodontal disease is not treated with professional prophylaxis (teeth cleaning) and, in some cases, surgery, it can lead to moderate-to-advanced periodontitis and further destruction of the bone and gum tissue. Tooth loss may occur and teeth may have to be removed.

Research shows that cigarette, cigar, and pipe smokers have a higher prevalence of moderate-to-severe periodontitis and higher prevalence and extent of attachment loss and gum recession than nonsmokers. They also have a higher number of missing teeth than nonsmokers; and although their gums bleed less, it is most often because nicotine constricts blood vessels, not because their gums are healthier. In addition, tobacco smokers are more likely than nonsmokers to have calculus (hardened or calcified dental plaque) formation on their teeth, to have developed periodontal pockets, to have lost bone that supports teeth, and to have lost supporting tissue that attaches the tooth to the bone.

Tobacco use can also affect the success of periodontal treatment. Cigarette smoke contains over 4,800 chemicals, 69 of which are known to cause cancer. When a smoker lights a cigarette and inhales, these toxins are drawn into the lungs. From there, they enter the bloodstream, which delivers them to every cell throughout the body, which cannot defend itself from them.

Smoking also reduces the delivery of oxygen and nutrients to the gingival tissue, and it interferes with healing and makes smokers less likely to respond to treatment, lengthening the time it takes for treatments to work.

✤ It's A Fact!!

Recent studies have shown that tobacco use in the form of cigarette, cigar, or pipe smoking, as well as smokeless tobacco use, are significant risk factors in the development and progression of periodontal disease. In turn, research links periodontal disease to increased risk of heart disease, stroke, poorly controlled diabetes, respiratory disease, and premature babies.

Smokeless tobacco—tobacco or a tobacco blend that users chew, inhale, or suck rather than smoke—also contributes to gum disease. Studies have shown that about 7–27% of regular smokeless tobacco users have gum recession and may lose the bone around the teeth and experience tooth loss. In addition, smokeless tobacco causes leukoplakia, white patches that form on the site where the user holds the tobacco. Research has also linked chewing tobacco to dental caries (cavities).

If you are a tobacco user, consider if you have the most common symptoms of periodontal disease:

- Bleeding gums during brushing

- Red, swollen, or tender gums

- Gums that have pulled away from the teeth

- Persistent bad breath

- Pus between the teeth and gums

- Loose or separating teeth

- A change in the way your teeth fit together when you bite

- A change in the fit of partial dentures

If you have any of the periodontal symptoms listed above, please consider consulting your oral health care professional for a complete periodontal evaluation to determine if you have periodontal disease. Consider how important it is to stop smoking or stop using smokeless tobacco in order to prevent periodontal disease, as well as other diseases associated with tobacco use. If you are a smoker, please consult your physician regarding a tobacco cessation program. Your dental hygienist is another good source of information about smoking, how to find resources on quitting, and its effect on your oral and overall health. For more information about proper oral health care, as well as brushing-and-flossing instructions, please ask your registered dental hygienist, or visit www.adha.org.

Chapter 43

Peripheral Arterial Disease

What Is Peripheral Arterial Disease?

Peripheral arterial disease (PAD) occurs when plaque builds up in the arteries that carry blood to your head, organs, and limbs. Plaque is made up of fat, cholesterol, calcium, fibrous tissue, and other substances in the blood.

When plaque builds up in arteries, the condition is called atherosclerosis. Over time, plaque can harden and narrow the arteries. This limits the flow of oxygen-rich blood to your organs and other parts of your body.

PAD usually affects the legs, but also can affect the arteries that carry blood from your heart to your head, arms, kidneys, and stomach. This chapter focuses on PAD that affects blood flow to the legs.

Overview

Blocked blood flow to your legs can cause pain and numbness. It also can raise your risk of getting an infection in the affected limbs. It may be hard for your body to fight the infection.

If severe enough, blocked blood flow can cause tissue death (gangrene). In very serious cases, this can lead to leg amputation.

About This Chapter: Text in this chapter is excerpted from "Peripheral Arterial Diseases," National Heart Lung and Blood Institute, September 2008.

If you have leg pain when you walk or climb stairs, talk to your doctor. Sometimes older people think that leg pain is just a symptom of aging. However, the cause for the pain could be PAD. Tell your doctor if you're feeling pain in your legs and discuss whether you should be tested for PAD.

Outlook

If you have PAD, your risk for coronary artery disease, heart attack, stroke, and transient ischemic attack ("mini-stroke") is six to seven times greater than the risk for people who don't have PAD. If you have heart disease, you have a one in three chance of having blocked leg arteries.

Although PAD is serious, it's treatable. If you have the disease, it's important to see your doctor regularly and treat the underlying atherosclerosis.

PAD treatment may slow or stop disease progress and reduce the risk of complications. Treatments include lifestyle changes, medicines, and surgery or procedures. Researchers continue to explore new therapies for PAD.

Other Names For Peripheral Arterial Disease

- Atherosclerotic peripheral arterial disease
- Peripheral vascular disease
- Vascular disease
- Hardening of the arteries
- Claudication
- Poor circulation
- Leg cramps from poor circulation

Causes Of Peripheral Arterial Disease

The most common cause of peripheral arterial disease (PAD) is atherosclerosis. The exact cause of atherosclerosis isn't known.

> ♣ **It's A Fact!!**
>
> Smoking is the main risk factor for PAD. If you smoke or have a history of smoking, your risk for PAD increases four times. Other factors, such as age and having certain diseases or conditions, also increase your risk.

The disease may start when certain factors damage the inner layers of the arteries. These factors include the following:

- Smoking

- High amounts of certain fats and cholesterol in the blood

- High blood pressure

- High amounts of sugar in the blood due to insulin resistance or diabetes

When damage occurs, your body starts a healing process. The healing may cause plaque to build up where the arteries are damaged.

Over time, the plaque may crack. Blood cell fragments called platelets stick to the injured lining of the artery and may clump together to form blood clots.

The buildup of plaque or blood clots can severely narrow or block the arteries and limit the flow of oxygen-rich blood to your body.

Risks For Peripheral Arterial Disease

PAD affects 8 to 12 million people in the United States. African Americans are more than twice as likely as Caucasians to have PAD. The major risk factors for PAD are smoking, age, and having certain diseases or conditions.

Smoking

Smoking is more closely related to getting PAD than any other risk factor. Your risk for PAD increases four times if you smoke or have a history of smoking. On average, smokers who develop PAD have symptoms ten years earlier than nonsmokers who develop PAD.

Age

As you get older, your risk for PAD increases. Genetic or lifestyle factors cause plaque to build in your arteries as you age.

About five percent of U.S. adults who are older than 50 have PAD. Among adults aged 65 and older, 12 to 20% may have PAD. Older age combined with other risk factors, such as smoking or diabetes, also puts you at higher risk.

Diseases And Conditions

A number of diseases and conditions can raise your risk for PAD:

- Diabetes: One in three people who has diabetes and is older than 50 is likely to have PAD

- High blood pressure or a family history of it

- High blood cholesterol or a family history of it

- Heart disease or a family history of it

- Stroke or a family history of it

> ✤ **It's A Fact!!**
>
> Quitting smoking slows the progress of PAD. Smoking even one or two cigarettes a day can interfere with PAD treatments. Smokers and people who have diabetes are at highest risk for PAD complications, including gangrene (tissue death) in the leg from decreased blood flow.

Signs And Symptoms Of Peripheral Arterial Disease

At least half of the people who have peripheral arterial disease (PAD) don't have any signs or symptoms of it. Others may have a number of signs and symptoms.

Even if they don't have signs or symptoms, people aged 70 or older, aged 50 or older and have a history of smoking or diabetes, or younger than 50 and have diabetes and one or more risk factors for atherosclerosis should discuss with getting checked for PAD with their doctors.

Intermittent Claudication

People who have PAD may have symptoms when walking or climbing stairs. These may include pain, numbness, aching, or heaviness in the leg muscles. Symptoms also may include cramping in the affected leg(s) and in the buttocks, thighs, calves, and feet. Symptoms may ease after resting.

These symptoms are called intermittent claudication. During physical activity, your muscles need increased blood flow. If your blood vessels are narrowed or blocked, your muscles won't get enough blood. When resting, the muscles need less blood flow, so the pain goes away.

About ten percent of people who have PAD have claudication. This symptom is more likely in people who also have atherosclerosis in other arteries.

Other Signs And Symptoms

Other signs and symptoms of PAD include the following:

- Weak or absent pulses in the legs or feet
- Sores or wounds on the toes, feet, or legs that heal slowly, poorly, or not at all
- A pale or bluish color to the skin
- A lower temperature in one leg compared to the other leg
- Poor nail growth on the toes and decreased hair growth on the legs
- Erectile dysfunction, especially among men who have diabetes

Diagnosing Peripheral Arterial Disease

Peripheral arterial disease (PAD) is diagnosed based on your medical and family histories, a physical exam, and results from tests.

PAD often is diagnosed after symptoms are reported. An accurate diagnosis is important, because people who have PAD are at increased risk for coronary artery disease (CAD), heart attack, stroke, and transient ischemic attack ("mini-stroke"). If you have PAD, your doctor also may want to look for signs of these conditions.

Preventing Peripheral Arterial Disease

Taking action to control your risk factors can help prevent or delay peripheral arterial disease (PAD) and its complications.

✔ Quick Tip

If you smoke, quit. Smoking is more closely related to getting PAD than any other risk factor. Your risk for PAD increases four times if you smoke or have a history of smoking. Talk to your doctor about programs and products that can help you quit smoking.

Know your family history of health problems related to PAD. If you or someone in your family has this disease, be sure to tell your doctor.

Your risk for PAD increases four times if you smoke. Talk to your doctor about programs and products that can help you quit smoking.

Follow a healthy eating plan that's low in total fat, saturated fat, trans fat, cholesterol, and sodium (salt). Eat more fruits, vegetables, and low-fat dairy products. If you're overweight or obese, work with your doctor to create a reasonable weight-loss plan.

The National Heart, Lung, and Blood Institute's Therapeutic Lifestyle Changes (TLC) and Dietary Approaches to Stop Hypertension (DASH) are two examples of healthy eating plans. (Visit www.nhlbi.nih.gov for more information.)

Get regular physical activity. Physical activity can improve your fitness level and your health. Talk to your doctor about what types of activity are safe for you.

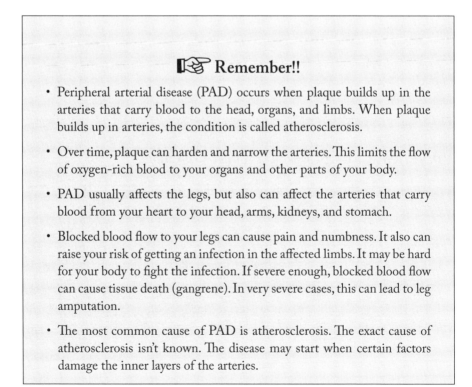

☞ Remember!!

- Peripheral arterial disease (PAD) occurs when plaque builds up in the arteries that carry blood to the head, organs, and limbs. When plaque builds up in arteries, the condition is called atherosclerosis.

- Over time, plaque can harden and narrow the arteries. This limits the flow of oxygen-rich blood to your organs and other parts of your body.

- PAD usually affects the legs, but also can affect the arteries that carry blood from your heart to your head, arms, kidneys, and stomach.

- Blocked blood flow to your legs can cause pain and numbness. It also can raise your risk of getting an infection in the affected limbs. It may be hard for your body to fight the infection. If severe enough, blocked blood flow can cause tissue death (gangrene). In very severe cases, this can lead to leg amputation.

- The most common cause of PAD is atherosclerosis. The exact cause of atherosclerosis isn't known. The disease may start when certain factors damage the inner layers of the arteries.

These lifestyle changes can reduce your risk for PAD and help prevent and control conditions that can lead to PAD, such as diabetes, high blood pressure, high blood cholesterol, heart disease, and stroke.

Living With Peripheral Arterial Disease

If you have peripheral arterial disease (PAD), you're also more likely to have coronary artery disease (CAD), heart attack, stroke, and transient ischemic attack (TIA, or "mini-stroke"). However, you can take steps to treat and control PAD and lower your risk for these other conditions.

If you have PAD, you may feel pain in your calf or thigh muscles after walking. Try to take a break and allow the pain to ease before walking again. Over time, this may increase the distance that you can walk without pain.

Talk with your doctor about taking part in a supervised exercise program. This type of program has been shown to reduce PAD symptoms.

- The major risk factors for PAD are smoking, age, and having certain medical conditions. Smoking is more closely related to getting PAD than any other risk factor. Your risk for PAD increases four times if you smoke.

- At least half of the people who have PAD don't have any signs or symptoms of it. Some people who have PAD may have symptoms when walking or climbing stairs. These may include pain, numbness, aching, or heaviness in the leg muscles. Symptoms also may include cramping in the legs, buttocks, thighs, calves, and feet.

- PAD is diagnosed based on your medial and family histories, a physical exam, and results from various tests. An accurate diagnosis is important, because people who have PAD are at increased risk for coronary artery disease, heart attack, stroke, and transient ischemic attack. If you have PAD, your doctor also may want to look for signs of these conditions.

- Treatments for PAD include lifestyle changes, medicines, and surgery or procedures. Treatment is based on your signs and symptoms, risk factors, and results from a physical exam and tests.

- Taking action to control your risk factors can help prevent or delay PAD and its complications.

Check your feet and toes regularly for sores or possible infections. Wear comfortable shoes that fit well. Maintain good foot hygiene and have professional medical treatment for corns, bunions, or calluses.

Ongoing Health Care Needs And Lifestyle Changes

See your doctor for checkups as he or she advises. If you have PAD, but don't have symptoms, you should still see your doctor regularly. Take all medicines as your doctor prescribes.

Lifestyle changes can help prevent or delay PAD and other related problems, such as CAD, heart attack, stroke, and TIA. Lifestyle changes include quitting smoking, controlling risk factors, getting regular physical activity, and following a healthy eating plan.

Chapter 44

Pregnancy Complications

Smoking During Pregnancy

Smoking is a major public health problem. All smokers face an increased risk of lung cancer, other lung diseases, and cardiovascular and other disorders. Smoking during pregnancy can harm the health of both a woman and her unborn baby. Currently, at least ten percent of women in the United States smoke during pregnancy.

In the United States and in other industrialized countries, 18% of women smoke. This proportion is somewhat smaller in developing countries where only eight percent of women smoke. Statistics from the United States are compelling. According to the U.S. Public Health Service, if all pregnant women in this country stopped smoking, there would be an estimated:

- 11% reduction in stillbirths, and

- 5% reduction in newborn deaths.

Cigarette smoke contains more than 2,500 chemicals. It is not known for certain which of these chemicals are harmful to the developing baby, but both nicotine and carbon monoxide play a role in causing adverse pregnancy outcomes.

How can smoking harm the newborn?

Smoking nearly doubles a woman's risk of having a low-birthweight baby. In 2004, 11.9% of babies born to smokers in the United States were of low birthweight (less than 5½ pounds), compared to 7.2% of babies of nonsmokers. Low birthweight can result from poor growth before birth, preterm delivery, or a combination of both. Smoking has long been known to slow fetal growth. Smoking also increases the risk of preterm delivery (before 37 weeks of gestation). Premature and low-birthweight babies face an increased risk of serious health problems during the newborn period, chronic lifelong disabilities (such as cerebral palsy, mental retardation and learning problems), and even death.

❖ It's A Fact!!

Pregnancy Complications

- Women who smoke have a greater risk for ectopic pregnancy and miscarriage.

Effects On The Unborn Child

- Smoking during pregnancy increases the risk for stillbirth, prematurity, and low birth weight in their babies.

- Women who smoke during pregnancy have lower levels of folate, a B vitamin that is important for preventing birth defects.

- Children of mothers who smoke during pregnancy may also be at increased risk for obesity and diabetes.

- A new study published in July 2008 found a definite connection between smoking in the first trimester of pregnancy and an increased risk of having a baby with cleft lip (a split lip that has not closed during the fetus' development).

- Some women have particular genes that may make them especially likely to deliver low birth weight infants if they smoke, although newborns of all female smokers have a greater risk for low weight. The good news is that women who stop smoking before becoming pregnant, or even during the first trimester, reduce the risk for a low birth weight baby to that of women who never smoked.

Source: "Smoking," © 2010 A.D.A.M, Inc. Reprinted with permission.

The more a pregnant woman smokes, the greater her risk of having a low-birthweight baby. However, if a woman stops smoking even by the end of her second trimester of pregnancy, she is no more likely to have a low-birthweight baby than a woman who never smoked.

A recent study suggests that women who smoke anytime during the month before pregnancy to the end of the first trimester are more likely to have a baby with birth defects, particularly congenital heart defects. The risk of heart defects appears to increase with the number of cigarettes a woman smokes.

Can smoking cause pregnancy complications?

Smoking is associated with a number of pregnancy complications. Smoking cigarettes doubles a woman's risk of developing placental problems. These include:

- Placenta previa (a low-lying placenta that covers part or all of the opening of the uterus), and

- Placental abruption (in which the placenta peels away, partially or almost completely, from the uterine wall before delivery).

Both can result in heavy bleeding during delivery that can endanger mother and baby, although cesarean delivery can prevent most deaths.

Smoking in pregnancy increases a woman's risk of premature rupture of the membranes (PROM), when the sac that holds the baby inside the uterus breaks before completion of 37 weeks of pregnancy. (Usually, when it breaks, normal labor ensues within a few hours.) If the rupture occurs before 37 weeks of pregnancy, it often results in the birth of a premature baby.

Does smoking affect fertility?

Cigarette smoking can cause reproductive problems before a woman even becomes pregnant. Studies show that women who smoke may have more trouble conceiving than nonsmokers. Studies suggest that fertility returns to normal after a woman stops smoking.

Does smoking during pregnancy cause other problems in babies or young children?

A 2003 study suggests that babies of mothers who smoke during pregnancy undergo withdrawal-like symptoms similar to those seen in babies of mothers who use some illicit drugs. For example, babies of smokers appear to be more jittery and difficult to soothe than babies of nonsmokers.

Babies whose mothers smoked during pregnancy are up to three times as likely to die from sudden infant death syndrome (SIDS) as babies of nonsmokers.

Can exposure to secondhand smoke during pregnancy harm the baby?

Studies suggest that babies of women who are regularly exposed to secondhand smoke during pregnancy may have reduced growth and may be more likely to be born with low birthweight. Pregnant women should avoid exposure to other people's smoke.

How can a woman stop smoking?

The March of Dimes recommends that women stop smoking before they become pregnant and do not smoke throughout pregnancy and after the baby is born. A woman's health care provider can refer her to a smoking-cessation program or suggest other ways to help her quit. The March of Dimes supports

---

✤ It's A Fact!!

Many studies have established that a pregnant woman's smoking raises her child's risk of disruptive behavior disorders and of delinquency in the teen and young adult years, but its behavioral effects in early life have been difficult to trace. Now, however, researchers funded by the National Institute on Drug Abuse have revealed associations between a child's in utero exposure to smoking and specific patterns of aberrant behavior as a toddler, at school age, and as a teen. The researchers propose that these patterns form a continuum, united by an underlying theme of disrupted social information processing

Source: Excerpted from "Behavioral Problems Related to Maternal Smoking during Pregnancy Manifest Early in Childhood," *NIDA Notes*, National Institute on Drug Abuse (NIDA), June 2008.

a 5- to 15-minute, 5-step counseling approach called "The 5 A's," which is performed by the health care provider during routine prenatal visits. This approach has been shown to improve smoking cessation rates among pregnant women by at least 30%. (Visit www.marchofdimes.com for more information.)

Studies suggest that certain factors make it more likely that a woman will be successful in her efforts to quit smoking during pregnancy. These include:

- Attempting to quit in the past
- Having a partner who doesn't smoke
- Getting support from family or other important people in her life
- Understanding the harmful effects of smoking

How does exposure to smoke after birth affect a baby?

It is important to stay smoke-free after the baby is born. Parents should refrain from smoking in the home and should ask visitors to do the same. Babies who are exposed to smoke suffer from more lower-respiratory illnesses (such as bronchitis and pneumonia) and ear infections than do other babies. Babies who are exposed to their parents' smoke after birth also may face an increased risk of asthma and SIDS.

Smoking harms a mother's health, too. Smokers have an increased risk of lung and other cancers, heart disease, stroke and emphysema (a potentially disabling and, sometimes, deadly lung condition). Quitting smoking makes parents healthier and better role models for their children.

Does the March of Dimes fund research on the risks of smoking during pregnancy?

The March of Dimes has long supported research on the risks of smoking during pregnancy. In the 1970s, March of Dimes–supported research suggested that nicotine and carbon monoxide reduce the supply of oxygen to the baby, perhaps explaining how these chemicals in cigarette smoke reduce fetal growth.

In 2002, a March of Dimes grantee published a study that may shed light on why some women who smoke cigarettes during pregnancy have low-birth-weight babies and others do not. The researcher reported that pregnant women who smoke are more likely to have a premature or low-birthweight baby if they have either of two common genetic traits (which influence the body's ability to dispose of certain chemicals). These findings could lead to better ways to identify and treat women at high risk of having a low-birthweight baby.

A current March of Dimes grantee is investigating whether smoking at a critical stage of embryonic palate development increases the risk of cleft lip/palate.

Chapter 45

Stroke

What is a stroke?

A stroke occurs when the blood supply to part of the brain is suddenly interrupted or when a blood vessel in the brain bursts, spilling blood into the spaces surrounding brain cells. In the same way that a person suffering a loss of blood flow to the heart is said to be having a heart attack, a person with a loss of blood flow to the brain or sudden bleeding in the brain can be said to be having a "brain attack."

Brain cells die when they no longer receive oxygen and nutrients from the blood or when they are damaged by sudden bleeding into or around the brain. Ischemia is the term used to describe the loss of oxygen and nutrients for brain cells when there is inadequate blood flow. Ischemia ultimately leads to infarction, the death of brain cells which are eventually replaced by a fluid-filled cavity (or infarct) in the injured brain.

When blood flow to the brain is interrupted, some brain cells die immediately, while others remain at risk for death. These damaged cells make up the ischemic penumbra and can linger in a compromised state for several hours. With timely treatment these cells can be saved.

About This Chapter: Text in this chapter is excerpted from "Stroke: Hope Through Research," National Institute of Neurological Disorders and Stroke (www.ninds.nih.gov), August 7, 2009.

Even though a stroke occurs in the unseen reaches of the brain, the symptoms of a stroke are easy to spot. They include sudden numbness or weakness, especially on one side of the body; sudden confusion or trouble speaking or understanding speech; sudden trouble seeing in one or both eyes; sudden trouble walking, dizziness, or loss of balance or coordination; or sudden severe headache with no known cause. All of the symptoms of stroke appear suddenly, and often there is more than one symptom at the same time. Therefore stroke can usually be distinguished from other causes of dizziness or headache. These symptoms may indicate that a stroke has occurred and that medical attention is needed immediately.

There are two forms of stroke: ischemic—blockage of a blood vessel supplying the brain, and hemorrhagic—bleeding into or around the brain.

✔ **Quick Tip**

How do you recognize stroke symptoms?

Symptoms of stroke appear suddenly. Watch for these symptoms and be prepared to act quickly for yourself or on behalf of someone you are with:

- Sudden numbness or weakness of the face, arm, or leg, especially on one side of the body.

- Sudden confusion, trouble talking, or understanding speech.

- Sudden trouble seeing in one or both eyes.

- Sudden trouble walking, dizziness, or loss of balance or coordination.

- Sudden severe headache with no known cause.

If you suspect you or someone you know is experiencing any of these symptoms indicative of a stroke, do not wait. Call 911 emergency immediately. There are now effective therapies for stroke that must be administered at a hospital, but they lose their effectiveness if not given within the first three hours after stroke symptoms appear. Every minute counts.

Who is at risk for stroke?

Some people are at a higher risk for stroke than others. Unmodifiable risk factors include age, gender, race/ethnicity, and stroke family history. In contrast, other risk factors for stroke, like high blood pressure or cigarette smoking, can be changed or controlled by the person at risk.

Unmodifiable Risk Factors: It is a myth that stroke occurs only in elderly adults. In actuality, stroke strikes all age groups, from fetuses still in the womb to centenarians. It is true, however, that older people have a higher risk for stroke than the general population and that the risk for stroke increases with age. For every decade after the age of 55, the risk of stroke doubles, and two-thirds of all strokes occur in people over 65 years old. People over 65 also have a seven-fold greater risk of dying from stroke than the general population. And the incidence of stroke is increasing proportionately with the increase in the elderly population. When the baby boomers move into the over-65 age group, stroke and other diseases will take on even greater significance in the health care field.

Gender also plays a role in risk for stroke. Men have a higher risk for stroke, but more women die from stroke. The stroke risk for men is 1.25 times that for women. But men do not live as long as women, so men are usually younger when they have their strokes and therefore have a higher rate of survival than women. In other words, even though women have fewer strokes than men, women are generally older when they have their strokes and are more likely to die from them.

Stroke seems to run in some families. Several factors might contribute to familial stroke risk. Members of a family might have a genetic tendency for stroke risk factors, such as an inherited predisposition for hypertension or diabetes. The influence of a common lifestyle among family members could also contribute to familial stroke.

The risk for stroke varies among different ethnic and racial groups. The incidence of stroke among African-Americans is almost double that of white Americans, and twice as many African-Americans who have a stroke die from the event compared to white Americans. African-Americans between the ages of 45 and 55 have four to five times the stroke death rate of whites. After age 55 the stroke mortality rate for whites increases and is equal to that of African-Americans.

Compared to white Americans, African-Americans have a higher incidence of stroke risk factors, including high blood pressure and cigarette smoking. African-Americans also have a higher incidence and prevalence of some genetic diseases, such as diabetes and sickle cell anemia, that predispose them to stroke.

Hispanics and Native Americans have stroke incidence and mortality rates more similar to those of white Americans. In Asian-Americans stroke incidence and mortality rates are also similar to those in white Americans, even though Asians in Japan, China, and other countries of the Far East have significantly higher stroke incidence and mortality rates than white Americans. This suggests that environment and lifestyle factors play a large role in stroke risk.

What are other stroke risk factors?

The most important risk factors for stroke are hypertension, heart disease, diabetes, and cigarette smoking. Others include heavy alcohol consumption, high blood cholesterol levels, illicit drug use, and genetic or congenital conditions, particularly vascular abnormalities. People with more than one risk factor have what is called "amplification of risk." This means that the multiple risk factors compound their destructive effects and create an overall risk greater than the simple cumulative effect of the individual risk factors.

Hypertension: Of all the risk factors that contribute to stroke, the most powerful is hypertension, or high blood pressure. People with hypertension have a risk for stroke that is four to six times higher than the risk for those without hypertension. One-third of the adult U.S. population, about 50 million people (including 40–70% of those over age 65) have high blood pressure. Forty to 90% of stroke patients have high blood pressure before their stroke event.

Heart Disease: After hypertension, the second most powerful risk factor for stroke is heart disease, especially a condition known as atrial fibrillation. Atrial fibrillation is irregular beating of the left atrium, or left upper chamber, of the heart. In people with atrial fibrillation, the left atrium beats up to four times faster than the rest of the heart. This leads to an irregular flow of blood and the occasional formation of blood clots that can leave the heart and travel to the brain, causing a stroke.

✤ It's A Fact!!

The "Stroke Belt"

Several decades ago, scientists and statisticians noticed that people in the southeastern United States had the highest stroke mortality rate in the country. They named this region the stroke belt. For many years, researchers believed that the increased risk was due to the higher percentage of African-Americans and an overall lower socioeconomic status (SES) in the southern states. A low SES is associated with an overall lower standard of living, leading to a lower standard of health care and therefore an increased risk of stroke. But researchers now know that the higher percentage of African-Americans and the overall lower SES in the southern states does not adequately account for the higher incidence of, and mortality from, stroke in those states. This means that other factors must be contributing to the higher incidence of and mortality from stroke in this region.

Recent studies have also shown that there is a stroke buckle in the stroke belt. Three southeastern states, North Carolina, South Carolina, and Georgia, have an extremely high stroke mortality rate, higher than the rate in other stroke belt states and up to two times the stroke mortality rate of the United States overall. The increased risk could be due to geographic or environmental factors or to regional differences in lifestyle, including higher rates of cigarette smoking and a regional preference for salty, high-fat foods.

Blood Cholesterol Levels: Most people know that high cholesterol levels contribute to heart disease. But many don't realize that a high cholesterol level also contributes to stroke risk. Cholesterol, a waxy substance produced by the liver, is a vital body product. It contributes to the production of hormones and vitamin D and is an integral component of cell membranes. The liver makes enough cholesterol to fuel the body's needs and this natural production of cholesterol alone is not a large contributing factor to atherosclerosis, heart disease, and stroke. Research has shown that the danger from cholesterol comes from a dietary intake of foods that contain high levels of cholesterol. Foods high in saturated fat and cholesterol, like meats, eggs, and dairy products, can increase the amount of total cholesterol in the body to alarming levels, contributing to the risk of atherosclerosis and thickening of the arteries.

Diabetes: Diabetes is another disease that increases a person's risk for stroke. People with diabetes have three times the risk of stroke compared to people without diabetes. The relative risk of stroke from diabetes is highest in the fifth and sixth decades of life and decreases after that. Like hypertension, the relative risk of stroke from diabetes is highest for men at an earlier age and highest for women at an older age. People with diabetes may also have other contributing risk factors that can amplify the overall risk for stroke. For example, the prevalence of hypertension is 40% higher in the diabetic population compared to the general population.

What are modifiable lifestyle risk factors?

Cigarette smoking is the most powerful modifiable stroke risk factor. Smoking is directly responsible for a greater percentage of the total number of strokes in young adults than in older adults. Risk factors other than smoking—like hypertension, heart disease, and diabetes—account for more of the total number of strokes in older adults.

Smoking increases the risk of stroke by promoting atherosclerosis and increasing the levels of blood-clotting factors, such as fibrinogen. In addition to promoting conditions linked to stroke, smoking also increases the damage that results from stroke by weakening the endothelial wall of the cerebro-vascular system. This leads to greater damage to the brain from events that occur in the secondary stage of stroke.

❖ It's A Fact!!

Smoking almost doubles a person's risk for ischemic stroke, independent of other risk factors, and it increases a person's risk for subarachnoid hemorrhage by up to 3.5%.

Heavy smokers are at greater risk for stroke than light smokers. The relative risk of stroke decreases immediately after quitting smoking, with a major reduction of risk seen after two to four years. Unfortunately, it may take several decades for a former smoker's risk to drop to the level of someone who never smoked.

High alcohol consumption is another modifiable risk factor for stroke. Generally, an increase in alcohol consumption leads to an increase in blood pressure. While scientists agree that heavy drinking is a risk for both hemorrhagic and ischemic stroke, in several research studies daily consumption of smaller amounts of alcohol has been found to provide a protective influence against ischemic stroke, perhaps because alcohol decreases the clotting ability of platelets in the blood. Moderate alcohol consumption may act in the same way as aspirin to decrease blood clotting and prevent ischemic stroke. Heavy alcohol consumption, though, may seriously deplete platelet numbers and compromise blood clotting and blood viscosity, leading to hemorrhage. In addition, heavy drinking or binge drinking can lead to a rebound effect after the alcohol is purged from the body. The consequences of this rebound effect are that blood viscosity (thickness) and platelet levels skyrocket after heavy drinking, increasing the risk for ischemic stroke.

The use of illicit drugs, such as cocaine and crack cocaine, can cause stroke. Cocaine may act on other risk factors, such as hypertension, heart disease, and vascular disease, to trigger a stroke. It decreases relative cerebrovascular blood flow by up to 30%, causes vascular constriction, and inhibits vascular relaxation, leading to narrowing of the arteries. Cocaine also affects the heart, causing arrhythmias and rapid heart rate that can lead to the formation of blood clots.

Marijuana smoking may also be a risk factor for stroke. Marijuana decreases blood pressure and may interact with other risk factors, such as hypertension and cigarette smoking, to cause rapidly fluctuating blood pressure levels, damaging blood vessels.

Other drugs of abuse, such as amphetamines, heroin, and anabolic steroids (and even some common, legal drugs, such as caffeine and L-asparaginase and pseudoephedrine found in over-the-counter decongestants), have been suspected of increasing stroke risk. Many of these drugs are vasoconstrictors, meaning that they cause blood vessels to constrict and blood pressure to rise.

What special risks do women face?

Some risk factors for stroke apply only to women. Primary among these are pregnancy, childbirth, and menopause. These risk factors are tied to hormonal fluctuations and changes that affect a woman in different stages of life. Research in the past few decades has shown that high-dose oral contraceptives, the kind used in the 1960s and 1970s, can increase the risk of stroke in women. Fortunately, oral contraceptives with high doses of estrogen are no longer used and have been replaced with safer and more effective oral contraceptives with lower doses of estrogen. Some studies have shown the newer low-dose oral contraceptives may not significantly increase the risk of stroke in women.

Other studies have demonstrated that pregnancy and childbirth can put a woman at an increased risk for stroke. Pregnancy increases the risk of stroke as much as three to 13 times. Of course, the risk of stroke in young women of child-bearing years is very small to begin with, so a moderate increase in risk during pregnancy is still a relatively small risk. Pregnancy and childbirth cause strokes in approximately eight in 100,000 women. Unfortunately, 25% of strokes during pregnancy end in death, and hemorrhagic strokes, although rare, are still the leading cause of maternal death in the United States. Subarachnoid hemorrhage, in particular, causes one to five maternal deaths per 10,000 pregnancies.

Are children at risk for stroke?

The young have several risk factors unique to them. Young people seem to suffer from hemorrhagic strokes more than ischemic strokes, a significant difference from older age groups where ischemic strokes make up the majority of stroke cases. Hemorrhagic strokes represent 20% of all strokes in the United States and young people account for many of these.

The symptoms of stroke in children are different from those in adults and young adults. A child experiencing a stroke may have seizures, a sudden loss of speech, a loss of expressive language (including body language and gestures), hemiparesis (weakness on one side of the body), hemiplegia (paralysis on one side of the body), dysarthria (impairment of speech), convulsions, headache, or fever. It is a medical emergency when a child shows any of these symptoms.

Most children who experience a stroke will do better than most adults after treatment and rehabilitation. This is due in part to the immature brain's great plasticity, the ability to adapt to deficits and injury. Children who experience seizures along with stroke do not recover as well as children who do not have seizures. Some children may experience residual hemiplegia, though most will eventually learn how to walk.

What disabilities can result from a stroke?

Although stroke is a disease of the brain, it can affect the entire body. Some of the disabilities that can result from a stroke include paralysis, cognitive deficits, speech problems, emotional difficulties, daily living problems, and pain.

- Paralysis

- Cognitive deficits

- Language deficits

- Emotional deficits

- Pain

Stroke is the number one cause of serious adult disability in the United States. Stroke disability is devastating to the stroke patient and family, but therapies are available to help rehabilitate post-stroke patients.

Speech and language problems arise when brain damage occurs in the language centers of the brain. Due to the brain's great ability to learn and change (called brain plasticity), other areas can adapt to take over some of the lost functions. Speech language pathologists help stroke patients relearn language and speaking skills, including swallowing, or learn other forms of communication. Speech therapy is appropriate for any patients with problems understanding speech or written words, or problems forming speech. A speech therapist helps stroke patients help themselves by working to improve language skills, develop alternative ways of communicating, and develop coping skills to deal with the frustration of not being able to communicate fully. With time and patience, a stroke survivor should be able to regain some, and sometimes all, language and speaking abilities.

❖ It's A Fact!!

Many stroke patients require psychological or psychiatric help after a stroke. Psychological problems, such as depression, anxiety, frustration, and anger, are common post-stroke disabilities. Talk therapy, along with appropriate medication, can help alleviate some of the mental and emotional problems that result from stroke. Sometimes it is also beneficial for family members of the stroke patient to seek psychological help as well.

What stroke therapies are available?

Physicians have a wide range of therapies to choose from when determining a stroke patient's best therapeutic plan. The type of stroke therapy a patient should receive depends upon the stage of disease. Generally there are three treatment stages for stroke: prevention, therapy immediately after stroke, and post-stroke rehabilitation. Therapies to prevent a first or recurrent stroke are based on treating an individual's underlying risk factors for stroke, such as hypertension, atrial fibrillation, and diabetes, or preventing the widespread formation of blood clots that can cause ischemic stroke in everyone, whether or not risk factors are present. Acute stroke therapies try to stop a stroke while it is happening by quickly dissolving a blood clot causing the stroke or by stopping the bleeding of a hemorrhagic stroke. The purpose of post-stroke rehabilitation is to overcome disabilities that result from stroke damage.

Therapies for stroke include medications, surgery, or rehabilitation.

Chapter 46

Sexual Health

Smoking And Sexual Health

The classic movie image of the post-sex cigarette makes it seem like smoking and sex are a natural fit. But smoking can wreak havoc on the reproductive system and on sexual health. If the threats of lung cancer, heart failure, and emphysema aren't enough to make you stuff the puff, check out what smoking can do to your sexual health.

For Her

Birth Control

Smoking and using combined hormonal contraception—the pill, the patch, the ring—can be risky. The older the woman is and the more she smokes, the greater the danger. In fact, women 35 and older who smoke are 10 times more likely to have a heart attack than those who don't smoke. Younger women who smoke may use combined hormonal methods, but they need to be very clear with the prescribing health care provider that they smoke.

The Menstrual Cycle

Some evidence indicates that smoking can affect a woman's menstrual cycle. Women who smoke may be more likely to have painful and irregular periods, and menstrual pain seems to last longer for smokers. When women quit smoking, they experience less menstrual irregularity.

Cervical Cancer And Orgasm

Cigarette smoking increases the risk of cervical cancer, and surgery for cervical cancer may interfere with orgasm.

Future Fertility

Most teen girls don't want to get pregnant now. But girls who smoke when they're teenagers may be hurting their chances of getting pregnant in the future. Some of the substances found in cigarettes can harm the ovaries, and women who smoke or have smoked in the past may have trouble getting pregnant.

Pregnancy

Here's something else to keep in mind for the future: smoking during pregnancy puts both the woman and her fetus at risk for health problems. Not only does smoking increase the woman's risk for serious complications during pregnancy and childbirth, but smoking during pregnancy is the largest preventable cause of both fetal and infant health risks and death. A woman who smokes may be at increased risk for ectopic pregnancy—when a fertilized egg implants somewhere outside of the uterus, usually in one of the fallopian tubes. Surgery is often needed to remove the embryo and possibly the damaged fallopian tube.

Smoking during pregnancy increases the risk of miscarriage. And women who smoke are more likely to have low birth-weight babies, who are less healthy and have an increased risk of death. Stillbirth or the death of the newborn during the first four weeks of life is also more common among women who smoke while pregnant.

✤ It's A Fact!!

For smokers, the chances of conceiving are decreased by 10 to 40% each menstrual cycle, and the longer a woman smokes, the longer it will take for her to get pregnant. Even light smoking can have an impact. (But don't count on smoking to be a reliable method of birth control.)

Research also suggests that secondhand smoke can damage the health of a woman and the fetus, so having a partner who smokes is a health risk.

For Him

Impotence

There is substantial evidence that links smoking with difficulty getting or maintaining an erection. Although impotence is less common in teen guys than in older men, studies show that smokers are at least 50% more likely to become impotent than nonsmokers. The many toxins in cigarettes—especially carbon monoxide—can damage the circulatory system, making it difficult for blood to reach the penis, which is necessary for erection. Quitting smoking can reduce the risk for impotence.

Fertility

The toxins found in cigarettes can also affect the testes, where sperm is produced. Smoking affects both semen and sperm, reducing their quality and affecting sperm motility. Men who smoke also tend to have lower sperm counts than nonsmokers and have more malformed sperm. This can make conception difficult and may also put a fetus at risk of developing from genetic material that has been damaged by smoking.

Improving Your Sexual Health

While some people quit smoking cold turkey, others have success with different routes: joining a program that helps people quit smoking, talking to a doctor or clinician about prescribing medication to reduce cravings, or trying nicotine-substitute chewing gum or patches. And some succeed with "alternative" methods such as hypnosis.

In the meantime:

- Try saving the money you would have spent on cigarettes to buy something special.
- Exercise to release endorphins and distract yourself from cigarette cravings.
- Socialize with nonsmokers.

- Snack on low-calorie vegetables to keep your hands and mouth active.

- Keep a list of reasons you want to quit and look at it every day.

- Enlist your family and friends to help you.

- Practice deep breathing and relaxation.

- Chew sugarless gum.

- Drink cold water.

Although it can be a challenge, quitting smoking is one of the best things you can do to improve your sexual health.

Part Five

Tobacco Use Cessation

Chapter 47

How Can I Quit Smoking?

First, congratulate yourself. Just reading this chapter is a huge step toward becoming tobacco free. Many people don't quit smoking because they think it's too hard to do. They think they'll quit someday.

It's true, for most people quitting isn't easy. After all, the nicotine in cigarettes is a powerfully addictive drug. But with the right approach, you can overcome the cravings.

The Difficulty In Kicking The Habit

Smokers may have started smoking because their friends did or because it seemed cool. But they keep on smoking because they became addicted to nicotine, one of the chemicals in cigarettes and smokeless tobacco.

Nicotine is both a stimulant and a depressant. That means it increases the heart rate at first and makes people feel more alert (like caffeine, another stimulant). Then it causes depression and fatigue. The depression and fatigue— and the drug withdrawal from nicotine—make people crave another cigarette to perk up again. According to many experts, the nicotine in tobacco is as addictive as cocaine or heroin.

About This Chapter: "How Can I Quit Smoking?" September 2009, reprinted with permission from www.kidshealth.org. Copyright © 2009 The Nemours Foundation. This information was provided by KidsHealth, one of the largest resources online for medically reviewed health information written for parents, kids, and teens. For more articles like this one, visit www.KidsHealth.org, or www.TeensHealth.org.

But don't be discouraged; millions of Americans have permanently quit smoking. These strategies can help you quit, too.

Put it in writing: People who want to make a change often are more successful when they put it in writing. So write down all the reasons why you want to quit smoking, such as the money you will save or the stamina you'll gain for playing sports. Keep that list where you can see it, and add to it as you think of new reasons.

Get support: People whose friends and family help them quit are much more likely to succeed. If you don't want to tell your parents or family that you smoke, make sure your friends know, and consider confiding in a counselor or other adult you trust. And if you're having a hard time finding people to support you (if, say, all your friends smoke and none of them is interested in quitting), you might consider joining a support group, either in person or online.

More Strategies That Work

Set a quit date: Pick a day that you'll stop smoking. Tell your friends (and your family, if they know you smoke) that you're going to quit smoking on that day. Just think of that day as a dividing line between the smoking you and the new and improved nonsmoker you'll become. Mark it on your calendar.

✤ It's A Fact!!
What are the immediate benefits of quitting smoking?

The immediate health benefits of quitting smoking are substantial. Heart rate and blood pressure, which were abnormally high while smoking, begin to return to normal. Within a few hours, the level of carbon monoxide in the blood begins to decline. (Carbon monoxide, a colorless, odorless gas found in cigarette smoke, reduces the blood's ability to carry oxygen.) Within a few weeks, people who quit smoking have improved circulation, don't produce as much phlegm, and don't cough or wheeze as often. Within several months of quitting, people can expect significant improvements in lung function.

Source: Excerpted from "Quitting Smoking: Why to Quit and How to Get Help," National Cancer Institute (www.cancer.gov), August 17, 2007.

Throw away your cigarettes—all of your cigarettes: People can't stop smoking with cigarettes still around to tempt them. Even toss out that emergency pack you have stashed in the secret pocket of your backpack. Get rid of your ashtrays and lighters, too.

Wash all your clothes: Get rid of the smell of cigarettes as much as you can by washing all your clothes and having your coats or sweaters dry-cleaned. If you smoked in your car, clean that out, too.

Think about your triggers: You're probably aware of the situations when you tend to smoke, such as after meals, when you're at your best friend's house, while drinking coffee, or as you're driving. These situations are your triggers for smoking—it feels automatic to have a cigarette when you're in them. Once you've figured out your triggers, try these tips:

- Avoid these situations. For example, if you smoke when you drive, get a ride to school, walk, or take the bus for a few weeks. If you normally smoke after meals, make it a point to do something else after you eat, like read or call a friend.

- Change the place. If you and your friends usually smoke in restaurants or get takeout and eat in the car, suggest that you sit in the no-smoking section the next time you go out to eat.

- Substitute something else for cigarettes. It can be hard to get used to not holding something and having something in your mouth. If you have this problem, stock up on carrot sticks, sugar-free gum, mints, toothpicks, or even lollipops.

Physical And Mental Effects

Expect some physical symptoms: If you smoke regularly, you're probably physically addicted to nicotine and your body may experience some symptoms of withdrawal when you quit. These may include:

- headaches or stomachaches;
- crabbiness, jumpiness, or depression;
- lack of energy;
- dry mouth or sore throat;
- desire to pig out.

Luckily, the symptoms of nicotine withdrawal will pass—so be patient. Try not to give in and sneak a smoke because you'll just have to deal with the symptoms longer.

Keep yourself busy: Many people find it's best to quit on a Monday, when they have school or work to keep them busy. The more distracted you are, the less likely you'll be to crave cigarettes. Staying active is also a good way to make sure you keep your weight down and your energy up, even as you're experiencing the symptoms of nicotine withdrawal.

Quit gradually: Some people find that gradually decreasing the number of cigarettes they smoke each day is an effective way to quit. However, this strategy doesn't work for everyone—you may find you have to stop completely at once. This is known as "cold turkey."

> **✤ It's A Fact!!**
> **Does quitting smoking lower the risk of cancer?**
>
> Quitting smoking substantially reduces the risk of developing and dying from cancer, and this benefit increases the longer a person remains smoke free. However, even after many years of not smoking, the risk of lung cancer in former smokers remains higher than in people who have never smoked.
>
> The risk of premature death and the chance of developing cancer due to cigarettes depend on the number of years of smoking, the number of cigarettes smoked per day, the age at which smoking began, and the presence or absence of illness at the time of quitting. For people who have already developed cancer, quitting smoking reduces the risk of developing a second cancer.
>
> Source: Excerpted from "Quitting Smoking: Why to Quit and How to Get Help," National Cancer Institute (www.cancer.gov), August 17, 2007.

Use a nicotine replacement if you need to: If you find that none of these strategies is working, you might talk to your doctor about treatments. Using a nicotine replacement, such as gum, patches, inhalers, or nasal sprays, can be very helpful. Sprays and inhalers are available by prescription only, and it's important to see your doctor before buying the patch and gum over the counter. That way, your doctor can help you find the solution that will work best for you. For example, the patch requires the least effort on your part, but it doesn't offer the almost instantaneous nicotine kick that gum does.

Slip-Ups Happen

If you slip up, don't give up: Major changes sometimes have false starts. If you're like many people, you may quit successfully for weeks or even months and then suddenly have a craving that's so strong you feel like you have to give in. Or maybe you accidentally find yourself in one of your trigger situations and give in to temptation.

If you slip up, it doesn't mean you've failed, it just means you're human. Here are some ways to get back on track:

Think about your slip as one mistake: Take notice of when and why it happened and move on.

- Did you become a heavy smoker after one cigarette? We didn't think so—it happened more gradually, over time. Keep in mind that one cigarette didn't make you a smoker to start with, so smoking one cigarette (or even two or three) after you've quit doesn't make you a smoker again.

✤ It's A Fact!!
What are the long-term benefits of quitting smoking?

Quitting smoking reduces the risk of cancer and other diseases, such as heart disease and lung disease, caused by smoking. People who quit smoking, regardless of their age, are less likely than those who continue to smoke to die from smoking-related illness. Studies have shown that quitting at about age 30 reduces the chance of dying from smoking-related diseases by more than 90%. People who quit at about age 50 reduce their risk of dying prematurely by 50% compared with those who continue to smoke. Even people who quit at about age 60 or older live longer than those who continue to smoke.

Source: Excerpted from "Quitting Smoking: Why to Quit and How to Get Help," National Cancer Institute (www.cancer.gov), August 17, 2007.

- Remind yourself why you've quit and how well you've done—or have someone in your support group, family, or friends do this for you.

Reward yourself: As you already know, quitting smoking isn't easy. Give yourself a well-deserved reward. Set aside the money you usually spend on cigarettes. When you've stayed tobacco free for a week, two weeks, or a month, buy yourself a treat like a new CD, book, movie, or some clothes. And every smoke-free year, celebrate again. You earned it.

Chapter 48

Smoking Cessation Tips

Quitting Is Hard

Nicotine is in all tobacco products. It makes you feel calm and satisfied, yet also alert and focused. But the more you smoke, the more nicotine you need to feel good. Soon, you don't feel "normal" without nicotine. This is nicotine addiction.

It takes time to break free from nicotine addiction. It may take more than one try to quit for good. Many ex-smokers say quitting was the hardest thing they ever did. So don't give up too soon. You will feel good again.

Quitting isn't easy. Just reading this chapter won't do it. You may try to quit several times before you're finally done with cigarettes. But you will learn something each time you try. It takes willpower and strength to beat your addiction to nicotine. Remember that millions of people have quit smoking for good. You can be one of them.

Preparing To Quit

Think about why you want to quit. Decide for sure that you want to quit, and then promise yourself you'll do it. It's okay to have mixed feelings. Don't let that stop you. There will be times every day that you don't feel like quitting. You will have to stick with it anyway. Find reasons that are important to you, such as health

About This Chapter: Text in this chapter is excerpted and adapted from "Clearing the Air: Quit Smoking Today," National Cancer Institute, NIH Pub. No. 08-1647, October 2008.

reasons, to feel proud of yourself, to be a better role model, to feel more in control of your life, or to have more time and money.

Write down all the reasons you want to quit. Keep your list where you'll see it often. Good places for your list are where you used keep your cigarettes, in your wallet or purse, in your kitchen or room, or in your car. When you reach for a cigarette, find your list of reasons for quitting. It will remind you why you want to stop.

Understand what makes you want to smoke. You want to smoke because your body now relies on nicotine. When the amount of nicotine in your body runs low, it triggers a craving—a strong, almost uncontrollable urge—for another cigarette. You may feel jittery, short-tempered, or anxious when you haven't smoked. Your body wants nicotine.

Triggers—people, places, activities, and feelings you associate with smoking—also make you want to smoke. Your triggers might be hearing the sounds of a party, finishing a task, or smelling coffee. Whatever your triggers, they can make you crave a cigarette.

You can get prepared to quit smoking by thinking of ways to avoid some triggers and creating alternatives for others. You'll find that the urge to smoke only lasts a few minutes. Even if it lasts longer, it will go away, whether or not you smoke. Fighting the urge to smoke is easier if you try these suggestions:

✔ Quick Tip
Know Your Triggers

If you know your triggers, you have a head start on avoiding situations that tempt you to smoke. The following is a list of some common triggers. Maybe only a few apply to you. The point is to recognize all the situations that trigger your craving for a cigarette.

- Waking in the morning
- Drinking something
- Smelling a cigarette
- Being with other smokers
- Seeing someone smoke
- Taking a break
- Talking on the phone
- Checking e-mail
- Surfing the internet
- Watching TV
- Driving or being a passenger in a car
- After eating
- After completing a task
- Feeling stressed
- Feeling lonely, depressed, or bored
- Feeling angry, irritable, or impatient

- Take a deep breath

- Keep your hands busy—write, doodle, or hold a coin or pencil

- Put something else in your mouth, such as a toothpick, sugar-free lollipop, or celery stick

- Go places where smoking isn't allowed, such as a library or nonsmoking restaurant

- Hang out with people who don't smoke

Options For Quitting Smoking

With many quit methods to choose from, be aware that no single approach works best for everyone. And you may need to try more than one method before you quit for good. Some quit methods require a doctor's prescription. While others do not, it's always a good idea to discuss your plan to quit smoking with your doctor.

Cold Turkey

For some smokers, "going cold turkey" seems like the easiest way to quit: Just stop smoking and tell yourself you'll never light up again. This works for some smokers—usually those with the lowest level of nicotine dependence—but not many. Fewer than five percent of smokers can quit this way. Most people aren't prepared when smoking habits and withdrawal symptoms trigger an intense urge to smoke. Research shows that most smokers have more success with one of the assisted quit methods discussed below. These methods have been tested and all of them are included in the U.S. Public Health Service guidelines for treating tobacco use and dependence.

Over-The-Counter Medications

You don't need a prescription to buy certain medications that can improve your success with quitting. Nicotine replacement therapy (NRT) products—lozenges, gum, or a patch—provide nicotine to help reduce your craving for nicotine and withdrawal symptoms, if any. This allows you to focus on changing the behavior and habits that trigger your urge to smoke.

Prescription Medications

Your doctor can prescribe medications to help you quit smoking. Some—inhalers and nasal sprays—act much like nonprescription nicotine replacement therapy. Other medications do not contain nicotine and work in different ways to help reduce your urge to smoke.

Counseling And Group Support

Many smokers quit with support provided by individual counseling or group treatment. You can combine these therapies with over-the-counter or prescription medications. Counseling can help you identify and overcome situations that trigger the urge to smoke. Research shows that success rates for all quit methods are higher when they are combined with a support program that provides encouragement through regularly scheduled one-on-one or group meetings or quitlines.

Steps To Quitting

Set A Quit Date

Finding a time to quit isn't easy. Any time can be a good time to quit when you are ready to try. Some smokers like to pick a day that is meaningful to them, such as birthday, the first day of vacation, New Year's Day (January 1), Independence Day (July 4), World No Tobacco Day (May 31), or The Great American Smokeout (the third Thursday of each November).

Quitlines   ✔ Quick Tip

Quitlines are free, telephone-based counseling programs that are available nationwide. When you call a quitline, you are teamed with a trained counselor who can help you develop a strategy for quitting or help you stay on the program you have chosen. The counselor often provides material that can improve your chances of quitting. You can call the National Cancer Institute's Smoking Quitline at 877-44U-Quit (877-448-7848) or the National Quitline at 800-QUITNOW (800-784-8669). These are national quitlines that can help you anywhere in the United States.

If you prefer online help, you can also text-message experts on LiveHelp at www.smokefree.gov.

✔ Quick Tip

You can remember five important steps toward quitting for good by remembering the word START:

- S: Set a quit date.

- T: Tell family, friends, and coworkers you plan to quit.

- A: Anticipate and plan for the challenges you will face while quitting.

- R: Remove cigarettes and other tobacco products from your home, car, and workplace if you have a job.

- T: Talk to your doctor about getting help to quit.

It doesn't have to be a special day to quit, however. For many people, *today* is the day. You can choose any day to be your quit day. When you are ready to take the first step toward quitting, take it.

Tell Others

Quitting smoking is easier with the support of others. Tell your family, friends, and other important people in your life you plan to quit and how they can help you. Some people like to have others ask them how things are going, while some find it annoying. Tell the people you care about exactly how they can help you. Here are some ideas:

- Ask everyone to understand if you have a change in mood; assure them it won't last long.

- Ask smokers who are close to you to quit with you or at least not smoke around you.

- Tell yourself and others: "The longer I go without cigarettes, the sooner I'll feel better."

- Tell yourself and others: "The worst withdrawal symptoms from smoking—irritability and trouble sleeping—may be over within two weeks."

Anticipate Challenges

Expecting challenges is an important part of getting ready to quit. Most people who have a hard time quitting and resume smoking do so in the first three months after trying to quit. Difficulty quitting is often caused by withdrawal symptoms—the physical discomfort smokers feel when they give up nicotine. It is your body's way of telling you it is learning to be nicotine-free. These feelings will go away in time.

Even as your physical withdrawal is decreasing, you may still be tempted to smoke when you feel stressed or down. Although it's a challenge to be ready for these times, knowing that certain feelings can trigger a craving to smoke will help you handle the tough times.

To understand your short- and long-term challenges, start by examining your smoking habits. Keeping a smoking journal can help you track how many cigarettes you smoke a day and what you are doing when you light up. Check for patterns in your smoking. You may find triggers you aren't even aware of. Perhaps cigarettes you smoke at certain times or circumstances mean different things to you. Some may be more important than others. Understanding what tempts you to smoke in the short and long term will help you control the urge to smoke before it hits.

Keep your journal with you so you can easily use it. Be sure to record the time you smoke, where you are, what you are doing, and what you are thinking or feeling. Rate how much you want the cigarette each time you smoke. Try this activity for at least a few days, making sure to record one day during the week and one day on the weekend. You may even find that the time you take to complete the journal helps you smoke less.

Remove Cigarettes And Other Tobacco Products From Your Environment

Getting rid of things that remind you of smoking also will help you get ready to quit. You should throw away all your tobacco supplies (cigarettes, lighters, matches, and ashtrays).Don't forget to check your drawers, coats, and bags. Make things clean and fresh in your home and car. Have your teeth cleaned and remove those nicotine stains.

✔ **Quick Tip**

When You Really Crave A Cigarette

Remember—the urge to smoke usually lasts only a few minutes. Try to wait it out. One reason it's important to get rid of all your cigarettes is to give yourself the time you need for these cravings to fade. Drink water or do something else until the urge passes. You also can use any of the tips below:

- Pick up something other than a cigarette: Try carrot or celery sticks, pickles, popsicles, sunflower seeds, apples, raisins, or pretzels

- Have a list of things you can do at a moment's notice: Organize your computer files, delete messages from your cell phone, or call a friend to chat

- Take a deep breath: Take ten slow, deep breaths and hold the last one. Then breathe out slowly. Relax.

- Clean something: Wash your hands or the dishes, vacuum, or clean out your car

- Make a move: Go outside or to a different room, or change what you are doing or who you are with.

No matter what, don't think, "Just one won't hurt." It will hurt. It will slow your progress toward your goal of being smoke-free. Remember—trying something to beat the urge is always better than trying nothing. The craving will go away.

Don't save the "just in case" pack of cigarettes! Saving one pack just makes it easier to start smoking again.

Talk To Your Doctor

It is important to tell your doctor when you are ready to quit. Your doctor can help you connect with the right resources to make your quit attempt successful. Remember—quitting "cold turkey" isn't your only choice.

Make sure to let your doctor or pharmacist know what medications you are taking. Nicotine changes how some drugs work. Your doctor may need to adjust some of your medications after you quit.

Big Day—Your Quit Date

So today is the big day—your quit date. Quitting is not easy, so to help you get through your first smoke-free days, we suggest that you keep busy and find new things to do, stay away from what tempts you, and plan to reward yourself.

Keep Busy

Keep busy today, spending as much time as you can in nonsmoking places. Create some new habits and mix up your daily routine. Today and the days ahead will be easier if you avoid things that remind you of smoking. Remember—it's harder to smoke if you are keeping yourself busy and finding new things to do. Here are some examples to get you started:

- Go to nonsmoking places: gyms, libraries, malls, museums, places of worship, smoke-free restaurants

- Be active: walk or run, take a bike ride, go for a swim, shoot hops, try a yoga class

- Distract your hands: hold something—a tennis ball, pen, or coin, squeeze Silly Putty®, knit or crochet, write a letter

- Drink the right stuff: avoid alcoholic drinks, drink a lot of water and low-sugar fruit juice, replace coffee or tea with a new healthy beverage

- Distract your mind: do a crossword puzzle, read a book, play cards

- Fool your mouth: try a toothpick or straw, eat a lollipop, chew sugar-free gum, eat carrot or celery sticks, brush your teeth often and use mouthwash

You may have a hard time concentrating in your early days as a nonsmoker. Mental activities, such as doing crossword puzzles or even reading a book or magazine, may be more challenging. Recognize that it may be difficult to stay mentally focused in the early stages of quitting. Remember—your skill in these activities will return.

Reward Yourself

Don't think of it as stopping smoking. Think of it as starting a new, healthier life style. Staying smoke-free is challenging. It takes some time. Be patient. You will begin to feel better. Set up rewards to remind yourself how hard you're working. For example, you could buy yourself something special to celebrate quitting or splurge on a massage or dinner at a new restaurant. You might want to go see a movie or sporting event or start a new hobby or exercise program.

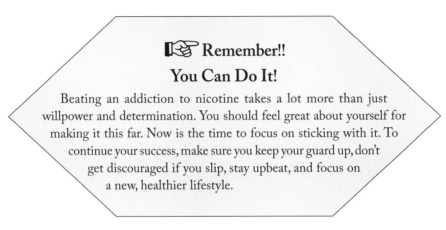

☞ Remember!!
You Can Do It!

Beating an addiction to nicotine takes a lot more than just willpower and determination. You should feel great about yourself for making it this far. Now is the time to focus on sticking with it. To continue your success, make sure you keep your guard up, don't get discouraged if you slip, stay upbeat, and focus on a new, healthier lifestyle.

Chapter 49

Putting A Stop To Smoky Thinking

It can be easy to lose sight of the benefits of quitting when a strong craving for a cigarette hits. When your body is asking for a cigarette, your mind may start to play tricks on you. Suddenly, it can be hard to think clearly—all of your good reasons for wanting to quit go up in smoke, and they are replaced by thoughts giving you permission to pick up that cigarette. There is no good reason to smoke. You know this. So if you are giving yourself a reason to smoke, you are probably experiencing an attack of smoky thinking.

Learning to recognize your smoky thinking is the key to beating it. Smoky thinking doesn't have to ruin your quit attempt, as long as you are ready to fight back with clear thinking. Look at the list below. Have you ever had these thoughts? If so, you have been a victim of smoky thinking! But with practice, next time you can be ready with a clear thinking response.

Smoky Thinking Thoughts And Clear Thinking Responses

- **Smoky Thinking:** I just need one cigarette to take the edge off these cravings.

About This Chapter: From "Putting a Stop to Smoky Thinking," produced by Smokefree Women, a project of the National Cancer Institute and other federal agencies (http://women.smokefree.gov), 2009.

- **Clear Thinking:** Cravings become weaker and less frequent with every day that I don't smoke. Even just one puff will feed the cravings and make them stronger.

- **Smoky Thinking:** It's been a long day. I deserve a cigarette.

- **Clear Thinking:** I deserve a reward after a long day, but there are better rewards than a cigarette. A favorite meal, a funny movie, or a hot shower will help me relax without ruining my quit attempt.

- **Smoky Thinking:** The urge to smoke is just too strong. I can't stand it.

- **Clear Thinking:** Even the strongest cravings last less than three minutes. The urge will go away whether I smoke or not, and smoking now will just make it even harder for me to quit later. I can find something else to do—anything—until the craving goes away.

- **Smoky Thinking:** I blew it. I smoked a cigarette. I might as well go ahead and finish the pack.

- **Clear Thinking:** I am still learning how to be a nonsmoker. It's normal to make some mistakes. But I don't have to smoke that next cigarette. I can learn from this mistake and keep going.

- **Smoky Thinking:** I can't deal with never being able to have another cigarette for the rest of my life. I only have to deal with today.

- **Clear Thinking:** Quitting happens one day at a time, sometimes one hour at a time! The future will take care of itself.

- **Smoky Thinking:** I am too cranky without my cigarettes. I am doing my friends and family a favor by smoking.

- **Clear Thinking:** My friends and family love me and understand that quitting smoking now is the best gift I can give them. Cranky or not, I am not doing them any favors by continuing to smoke.

- **Smoky Thinking:** I am doing really well. Just one cigarette won't hurt.

- **Clear Thinking:** I have never smoked just one before. One cigarette always leads to another. I don't want to undo all my progress by smoking a cigarette now.

- **Smoky Thinking:** It's too hard to quit smoking. I can't do this.

- **Clear Thinking:** Quitting and staying away from cigarettes is hard, but it's not impossible. About 40,000,000 Americans have quit smoking. If other people can do it, so can I. It is too important to give up on.

- **Smoky Thinking:** I've been smoking for so long; quitting won't make a difference now.

- **Clear Thinking:** No matter how long I've been smoking, my body will benefit from quitting. The healing process starts right away, and before long I will start to feel healthier and look better.

- **Smoky Thinking:** I know people who smoked their whole lives and never got sick.

- **Clear Thinking:** It's true that some people get lucky. But there is no way of knowing whether I will be one of the lucky ones, and I am not willing to risk my life. The only safe choice is to quit smoking now.

- **Smoky Thinking:** I have already cut down to a safe level.

- **Clear Thinking:** There is no safe level of smoking. Smoking less is a good first step, but there are many more benefits when I don't smoke at all. Plus, every cigarette that I smoke feeds the habit and makes it that much harder to quit.

Chapter 50

Nicotine Replacement Therapy

Nicotine replacement therapy involves the use of products that provide low doses of nicotine that do not contain the contaminants found in smoke. The goal of therapy is to relieve cravings for nicotine and ease the symptoms of withdrawal.

In general, nicotine replacement therapy benefits moderate-to-heavy smokers the most. However, it does appear somewhat helpful for light smokers (people who smoke fewer than 15 cigarettes a day).

Nicotine Patches: Nicotine patches deliver nicotine through the skin. This is called transdermal nicotine delivery. It is effective in reducing symptoms during withdrawal. Nicotine patches are available over the counter.

Patches may work in different ways:

- Step-Down Approach: Patches that use this method include NicoDerm CQ. The patches come in three strengths (21, 14, and 7 mg). You use the strongest dose first and reduce it gradually over a period of eight to ten weeks. A 21 mg patch is about equal to 15 cigarettes. A heavy smoker may need to wear two patches at first.

- Single-Step Approach. The single-step patch (Nicotrol) can be taken off after 16 hours and replaced eight hours later. It can be used for only six weeks.

About This Chapter: Text in this chapter is excerpted from "Smoking," © 2010 A.D.A.M, Inc. Reprinted with permission.

Patches are applied and used in similar ways:

- A single patch is worn each day and replaced after 24 hours.

- To avoid skin irritation it is applied to different hairless locations above the waist and below the neck each day.

- People can wear the patches for 24 hours, but some have reported odd dreams and have disliked the sensation of the patch during the night.

✤ It's A Fact!!

Myth: Nicotine replacement therapy (NRT) does not work.

Truth: NRT does work. NRT can double a smoker's chances of quitting smoking. The likelihood of staying quit for more than six months is increased when a smoker uses NRT according to the directions.

Myth: The nicotine in cigarettes is the same as the nicotine found in nicotine replacement therapy (NRT) products, so I'm just trading one addiction for another.

Truth: No, the products are different and the likelihood of long-term addiction to NRT is very low. The nicotine found in NRT is regulated by the Federal Drug Administration (FDA). The amount of nicotine in NRT is less than in cigarettes and it is delivered more slowly. NRT products have a much lower risk of addiction than cigarettes.

Myth: If I use NRT, I will experience no withdrawal symptoms or cravings from quitting smoking.

Truth: NRT does reduce withdrawal symptoms associated with cigarette smoking. However, it may not completely eliminate them. The symptoms most helped by NRT include: irritability, frustration, anger, craving, hunger, anxiety, difficulty concentrating, restlessness, and insomnia. NRT achieves the best results when combined with a personal quit plan.

Myth: NRT causes disease.

Truth: The effect of NRT on the body is not fully known, but NRT products are safer than cigarettes. The negative health effects of cigarettes are proven. Of the 4,000 chemicals found in tobacco smoke, over 60 are known to cause cancer.

People who wear the patch all the time, however, have fewer withdrawal symptoms and slightly better abstinence rates than those who take it off at night.

- Patches should be stored and discarded safely, particularly in homes with small children. Small children have been poisoned and gotten sick from wearing, chewing, or sucking on nicotine patches. There have been no reports of death from children who have been poisoned.

By using NRT to quit smoking you reduce your exposure to many chemicals found in tobacco smoke.

Myth: If I use one NRT product, I cannot use others.

Truth: No, NRT products can be used alone or in combination. Talk to your doctor before doing so.

Myth: NRT is too expensive.

Truth: Over time the cost of NRT is less expensive than the cost of cigarettes. NRT is generally used for a limited time, whereas cigarettes are typically consumed many years. Compare the price of the NRT products to the average price of $3.51 for a package of 20 cigarettes in South Carolina (lowest in the United States) and the $5.96 for a package of 20 cigarettes in Alaska. Here is a summary of average daily costs for NRT products:

- Nicotine Nasal Spray: $3.40
- Nicotine Patches: $3.91
- Nicotine Lozenges: $4.98
- Nicotine Gum: $5.81
- Nicotine Inhaler: $6.07

Myth: Only healthy people can use NRT.

Truth: Under the direction of your doctor most people can use NRT. Generally, NRT can be safely used by people with diabetes or high blood pressure and does not increase the risk of heart attacks.

Source: Excerpted from "Dispelling Myths about Nicotine Replacement Therapy," National Cancer Institute (http://www.smokefree.gov), 2007.

- The U.S. Food and Drug Administration (FDA) recommends using the patches for three to five months, although some studies suggest that using them for eight weeks achieves the maximum benefits.

- Children should not come in contact with the patches, even while the smoker is wearing them. If the child has worn the patch, the affected skin should be washed right away. Urgent medical care may be required if the child has eaten nicotine or worn a patch for a prolonged time.

Nicotine Gum: Nicotine gum (Nicorette) is available over the counter and has helped many people quit. Some prefer it to the patch because they can control the nicotine dosage, and chewing satisfies the oral urge associated with smoking.

Tips for using the gum:

- If you are just starting to quit, chew one to two pieces each hour. A smoker should not chew more than 20 pieces a day.

- The goal is to stop using the gum by six months, but about three percent of people continue to use it long after they have quit smoking.

- The gum must be chewed slowly until it develops a peppery taste. It is then tucked between the gum and cheek where it is stored so that the nicotine can be absorbed.

- Coffee, tea, soft drinks, and acidic beverages may interfere with nicotine absorption, so people should wait at least 15 minutes after drinking before chewing a piece of gum.

Some people prefer other methods or cannot use the gum for the following reasons:

- They find the taste of the gum unpleasant.

- Side effects specific to the gum may include upset stomach, mouth ulcers, hiccups, and throat irritation.

- They are embarrassed by chewing gum.

- They wear dentures.

Long-term dependence may be a problem with the gum. Although such dependence is probably safer than smoking, research is needed to confirm this, and experts recommend people chew gum for no more than six months.

The Nicotine Inhaler: The nicotine inhaler resembles a plastic cigarette holder. It comes with a number of nicotine cartridges, which are inserted into the inhaler and "puffed" for about 20 minutes, up to 16 times a day. The dose is gradually decreased. It requires a prescription in the United States. Several studies have reported that the inhaler triples abstinence rates (between 17 to 28%) compared with placebo (six to nine percent) after six months.

It has some specific advantages over other nicotine replacement products:

- The inhaler provides varying doses of nicotine on demand (as opposed to continuously with the patch or the gum) and is relatively fast acting. Blood nicotine levels peak about 20 minutes after using the inhaler, comparable to the gum and faster than the two to four hours seen with the patch.

- It satisfies oral urges.

- Most of the nicotine vapor is delivered in the mouth, not into the lung airways (although some people experience mouth or throat irritation and cough).

- Using a combination of the inhaler and the patch may be particularly effective.

The Nicotine Nasal Spray: The nasal spray satisfies immediate cravings by providing doses of nicotine rapidly and thus may play a useful role in conjunction with slower-acting nicotine replacement therapies. (Nicotine levels peak within five to ten minutes after administering the spray). The spray can irritate the nose, eyes, and throat, so it may not be suitable for those with allergies or sinus infections. Most people, however, can tolerate the side effects, which usually go away within the first few days.

Nicotine Lozenge: A nicotine lozenge (Commit) is available over the counter. It is made from pressed tobacco and comes in two strengths for heavier or lighter smokers. Side effects included heartburn, hiccups, nausea, headaches, and cough. The Commit lozenge also contains phenylalanine, a chemical that certain people may need to avoid.

Facts About Nicotine Replacement Therapy

- Not cheating on the very first day of nicotine-replacement use increases the chance of quitting permanently by tenfold.

- The more cigarettes a patient smokes, the higher the dose of nicotine replacement that may be required at the start.

- Adding a counseling program may boost the effect of any nicotine replacement program.

- Do not smoke while using nicotine replacement. It can cause nicotine to build up to toxic levels.

- Nicotine replacement helps prevent weight gain while it is being used, but people are still at higher risk for gaining weight when they stop all nicotine.

Side Effects: Side effects of any nicotine replacement product may include headaches, nausea, and other gastrointestinal problems. People often experience sleeplessness in the first few days, particularly with the patch, but the insomnia usually passes. Patients using very high doses are more likely to have symptoms. Reducing the dose can prevent them.

Special Concerns for Specific Individuals: There has been some concern that the patch might be harmful for people with heart or circulatory disease, but studies are finding that it poses no danger for these individuals. In fact, it may help reduce angina attacks brought on by exercise. However, unhealthy cholesterol levels (lower HDL levels) caused by smoking remain abnormal with use of the nicotine patch. HDL levels improve when all nicotine is stopped.

Nicotine replacement may not be completely safe in pregnant women, although it has been used successfully in this group without ill effect. There is an increase in heart rates in unborn children of women who use the patch as compared with those who smoke.

Keep all nicotine products away from children. Nicotine is a poison. All nicotine products should be kept safely away from small children. A parent should call a physician or a poison control center immediately if a child has been exposed to a nicotine replacement product, even for a short duration. Parents should also call

☞ Remember!!

Nicotine replacement therapy (NRT) helps individuals quit smoking by reducing the craving sensations associated with withdrawal from the nicotine in tobacco. NRT products provide controlled amounts of nicotine. Individuals reduce their use of NRT products over time, allowing their bodies to gradually adjust to increasingly lower nicotine levels.

- Nicotine patches are available over-the-counter. The nicotine patch is placed on the skin and supplies a small and steady amount of nicotine into the body. Nicotine patches contain varied concentrations of nicotine (21 mg, 14 mg, or 7 mg, for example) and the user reduces the dose over time.

- Nicotine gum is available over-the-counter. Nicotine gum is chewed to release nicotine that is absorbed through tissue inside the mouth. The user chews the gum until it produces a tingling feeling, then the gum is placed (parked) between the cheek and gum tissue. Nicotine gums have varied concentrations of nicotine (typically 2 mg or 4 mg) to allow the user to reduce the amount of nicotine in their system.

- Nicotine lozenges are available over-the-counter. Nicotine lozenges look like hard candy and are placed in your mouth to dissolve slowly. The nicotine lozenge (typically 2 mg or 4 mg dose of nicotine) releases nicotine as it slowly dissolves in the mouth.

- Nicotine inhalers are available by prescription only. A nicotine inhaler consists of a cartridge attached to a mouthpiece. Inhaling through the mouthpiece delivers a specific amount of nicotine to the user.

- Nicotine nasal sprays are available by prescription only. Nicotine nasal spray is a pump bottle containing nicotine that is inserted into the nose and sprayed. Nicotine nasal spray can be used for fast craving control, especially for heavy smokers.

Source: Excerpted and adapted from "Preparing to Quit: Medication Guide," National Cancer Institute (smokefree.gov), 2006.

the doctor if a small child has been exposed to a nicotine product and has any symptoms, including stomach upset, irritability, headaches, a rash, or fatigue.

Warnings Against Long-Term Use: No one should use nicotine replacement therapies as a long-term substitute for smoking. Any nicotine replacement therapy should be temporary. In one study, use of nicotine gum for more than a year was associated with insulin resistance, an abnormality that occurs in diabetes. Some studies have now suggested that nicotine itself may have properties that increase the risk for cancer, independent of carcinogenic chemicals in smoke. More studies are needed.

Chapter 51

Medications To Help You Quit Smoking

This information was assembled to provide you with a general understanding of the current medications used by smokers who are trying to quit. Please note that this chapter may not describe every product available. All of these medicines have been shown to be useful for helping smokers quit.

Dosing information provided in descriptions of these products is intended only to illustrate typical use of these medications. Individual dosing for prescription medications must be determined by a physician. If you are pregnant, breastfeeding, or have a severe medical problem, talk with your doctor before starting any new medication.

First Line Medications

- Bupropion
- Varenicline

Second Line Medications

- Nortriptyline
- Clonidine

About This Chapter: Text in this chapter is adapted from "Preparing to Quit: Medication Guide," "Bupropion Fact Sheet," "Varenicline Fact Sheet," "Nortriptyline Fact Sheet," and "Clonidine Fact Sheet," documents that are part of the *Online Guide to Quitting*, produced by the National Cancer Institute, 2006; available at http://smokefree.gov.

Facts About Bupropion

Bupropion, also known as Zyban, is a prescription medication that helps to reduce nicotine withdrawal symptoms and the urge to smoke. Bupropion can be used safely with nicotine replacement products.

✔ **Quick Tip**
There is no one best medicine for all smokers. Always read the instructions on the package carefully and talk with your doctor or pharmacist if you have questions.

Dosing: Take 150 mg every morning for three days. Then increase to 150 mg twice daily for seven to 12 weeks. Unlike NRT products, smokers should begin treatment with bupropion one to two weeks before they quit smoking. For maintenance therapy, smokers can take 150 mg twice daily for up to six months.

Side Effects: Side effects may include dry mouth, difficulty sleeping, headaches, dizziness, and skin rashes.

Precautions: Smokers who are pregnant or breastfeeding should try to quit first without assistance from bupropion. Bupropion should be used during pregnancy only if the associated benefits outweigh the associated risks.

Seizures: Smokers who have a history of seizure, cranial trauma, or severe hepatic impairment must use bupropion with extreme caution.

Facts About Varenicline

Varenicline, also known as Chantix, is a prescription medication that eases nicotine withdrawal symptoms and blocks the effects of nicotine from cigarettes if the user resumes smoking.

☞ **Remember!!**
This chapter provides general information it may not provide you with all the information you need to make the decision about using the medications that are discussed. Always read the instructions on the package carefully and talk with your doctor or pharmacist if you have questions. If you are pregnant, breastfeeding, or have a severe medical problem, talk with your doctor before starting any new medication.

Dosing: Users take one pill twice daily.

Side Effects: Side effects may include nausea, change in dreaming, constipation, gas, and vomiting. There have been rare reports of mood swings, depression and suicidal thoughts. Your doctor will want to monitor this carefully.

Precautions: Smokers who are pregnant or breastfeeding should try to quit first without assistance from varenicline. Varenicline should be used during pregnancy only if the associated benefits outweigh the associated risks.

Kidney Problems: Smokers should not use varenicline if they have kidney problems.

Facts About Nortriptyline

Description of Product: Nortriptyline, also known as Aventyl, is generally prescribed to treat depression; however nortriptyline has been prescribed to assist with smoking cessation when the first line medications do not work. The use of nortriptyline for smoking cessation has not yet been approved by the U.S. Food and Drug Administration (FDA).

Dosing: The first dose of nortriptyline is provided approximately 10–28 days before a quit attempt at a dose of 25 mg daily, increasing gradually to a target dose of 75–100 mg per day and continuing for 12 weeks.

Side Effects: Side effects may include drowsiness, dry mouth, lightheadedness, blurred vision, urinary retention, and tremor.

Precautions: Nortriptyline is not currently approved by the FDA for the treatment of nicotine addiction. Doctors sometimes prescribe these drugs to help people quit smoking when the first line of treatment does not help with cessation.

Facts About Clonidine

Clonidine, also known as Catapres, is generally prescribed to treat high blood pressure; clonidine may reduce tobacco withdrawal symptoms when first line medications do not work. The use of clonidine for smoking cessation has not yet been approved by the FDA.

Dosing: Clonidine dosages for tobacco cessation have ranged from 0.15 to 0.75 mg a day orally and 0.1 to 0.3 mg a day transdermally. Therapy is usually initiated at 0.1 mg orally twice daily or 0.1 mg a day transdermally and is increased by 0.10 mg a day each week as tolerated.

Side Effects: Side effects may include dry mouth, drowsiness, dizziness, sedation, and constipation.

Precautions: Clonidine is not currently approved by the FDA for the treatment of nicotine addiction. Doctors sometimes prescribe this drug to help people quit smoking when the first line of treatment does not help with cessation.

Chapter 52

Dealing With The Effects Of Nicotine Withdrawal

Handling Cravings... Without Smoking

Nicotine And Your Body And Mind

As a smoker, you are used to having a certain level of nicotine in your body. You control that level by how much you smoke, how deeply you inhale the smoke, and by the kind of tobacco you use. When you quit, cravings develop when the body wants more nicotine.

When you are exposed to smoking triggers or even when you use a small amount of nicotine, your mood changes, and cravings for tobacco can go up as well as your heart rate and blood pressure. Cravings are NOT "just in your head."

About This Chapter: This chapter includes text from the following fact sheets produced by the National Cancer Institute in November 2004: "Quitting Tobacco: Handling Cravings... Without Smoking," "Quitting Tobacco: Handling Irritability And Frustration... Without Smoking," "Quitting Tobacco: Handling Stress... Without Smoking," "Quitting Tobacco: Handling Anxiety... Without Smoking," "Quitting Tobacco: Handling Depression... Without Smoking," "Quitting Tobacco: Facing The Morning... Without Smoking," "Quitting Tobacco: Facing Boredom... Without Smoking," "Quitting Tobacco: Enjoying Coffee And Tea... Without Smoking," "Quitting Tobacco: Enjoying Meals... Without Smoking," "Quitting Tobacco: Driving Or Riding In A Car... Without Smoking," and "Quitting Tobacco: Being Around Other Smokers... Without Smoking." These fact sheets were adapted from material developed by the Tobacco Education and Prevention Program of the Arizona Department of Health Services and the Arizona Smokers' Helpline of the University of Arizona.

What To Expect

Cravings usually begin within an hour or two after you stop smoking, peak for several days, and may last several weeks.

The urge to smoke will come and go. Your cravings will be strongest in the first week after you quit using tobacco. Cravings usually last only a very brief period of time.

You may also experience cravings that follow each other in rapid succession. As the days pass, the cravings will get farther apart. There is some evidence that mild occasional cravings may last for six months.

What To Do

- Remind yourself that cravings will pass.
- As a substitute for smoking, try chewing on carrots, pickles, sunflower seeds, apples, celery, or sugarless gum or hard candy. Keeping your mouth busy may stop the psychological need to smoke.
- Try this exercise: Take a deep breath through your nose and blow out slowly through your mouth. Repeat 10 times.
- Avoid situations and activities (like drinking alcohol) that you normally associate with smoking.

Related Notes

Nicotine cravings may be reduced by using nicotine replacement products, which deliver small, steady doses of nicotine into the body.

Handling Irritability And Frustration... Without Smoking

What To Expect

- When you quit smoking, you may feel edgy and short-tempered.
- You may want to give up on tasks more quickly than usual.
- You may be less tolerant of others' behavior.
- You may get into more arguments.

✔ Quick Tip

How To Get Help

If you or someone you know wants help with giving up tobacco, please call the National Cancer Institute's Smoking Quitline toll-free at 877-44U-QUIT (877-448-7848). The information specialists on the Quitline can provide suggestions and support to help smokers break the habit.

The federal government's Smoke-free.gov website (http://www.smoke-free.gov/) allows you to choose the help that best fits your needs. You can get immediate assistance:

- View an online step-by-step cessation guide.
- Find state quitline telephone numbers.
- Instant message an expert through the National Cancer Institute's LiveHelp service.
- Download, print, or order publications about quitting smoking.

Did You Know?

Studies have found that most quitters report increased feelings of irritability, anger, and frustration within a week of quitting. If feelings of irritability, anger, and frustration occur, they usually begin on the first day, peak during the first couple of weeks, and disappear within a month.

What To Do

- Take a walk.
- Exercise.
- Reduce caffeine.
- Soak in a hot bath.
- Read up on relaxation/meditation techniques and use one.
- Take one minute and, with your eyes closed, pay attention to your breathing pattern. Breathe in deeply through your nose and breathe out through your mouth.

Nicotine And Your Body And Mind

When your body does not get nicotine, you may feel irritable, angry, and frustrated. Quitting will temporarily change your brain chemistry. These temporary changes may result in your experiencing negative emotions.

Related Notes

Feelings of anger, irritability, and frustration may be reduced by using nicotine replacement products, which deliver small, steady doses of nicotine into the body.

Handling Stress... Without Smoking

What To Expect

After you quit smoking, handling the normal stresses in your life may become more of a challenge. Quitting smoking itself is stressful and adds to your stress load.

Did You Know?

- Most smokers report that one reason they smoke is to handle stress.

- You may become more aware of stress during withdrawal. This happens because smoking cigarettes actually relieves some of your stress by releasing powerful chemicals in your brain.

- As you go longer without smoking, you will get better at handling stress, especially if you learn relaxation techniques.

Nicotine And Your Body And Mind

Everyday worries, responsibilities, and hassles can all contribute to stress. It is thought that once nicotine enters your brain, it stimulates production of a number of the brain's most powerful chemical messengers. These chemicals (epinephrine, norepinephrine, dopamine, arginine, vasopressin, beta-endorphin, and acetylcholine) are involved in alertness, pain reduction, learning, memory, pleasure, and the reduction of both anxiety and pain.

What To Do

- Know the causes of stress in your life (your job, your school, money).

- Identify the stress signals (headaches, nervousness, or trouble sleeping).

- Create peaceful times in your everyday schedule. (For example, set aside an hour where you can get away from other people and your usual environment.)

- Try new relaxation methods and stick with the best one for you.

- Rehearse and visualize your relaxation plan. Put your plan into action. Change your plan as needed.

- Seek and learn relaxation techniques such as progressive relaxation.

Related Notes

You may find it helpful to visit your library or bookstore to pick up a book about how to handle stress.

Handling Anxiety... Without Smoking

What To Expect

- You may feel quite tense and agitated within 24 hours of quitting.

- You may feel a tightness in your muscles—especially around the neck and shoulders.

- These feelings will pass with time.

Did You Know?

Recent studies have found that most quitters report feelings of increased anxiety within a week of quitting. If anxiety occurs, it will usually begin within the first day, peak in the first couple of weeks, and disappear within a month.

What To Do

- Take a walk.

- Take a hot bath.

- Try a massage.

- Try to take a few minutes out of your day to meditate, or do stretching exercises.

- Set aside some quiet time every morning and evening—a time when you can be alone in a quiet environment.

❖ It's A Fact!!

When you smoke, your brain chemistry changes temporarily so that you experience decreased anxiety, enhanced pleasure, and alert relaxation. This is why it feels good when you smoke.

Nicotine And Your Mind And Body

Anxiety is usually measured as an increase in muscle tension as well as an increased sensitivity to muscle tension. Laboratory research shows that the anxiety produced from quitting tobacco may be due to temporary changes in your brain chemistry.

Handling Depression... Without Smoking

What To Expect

It is normal to feel sad for a period of time after you first quit smoking. Many people have a strong urge to smoke when they feel depressed. If you give in to your craving for a cigarette, you may feel sad that you could not stick with your decision to quit.

Did You Know?

Having a history of depression is associated with more severe withdrawal symptoms—including more severe depression. Some studies have found that many people with a history of major depression will have a new major depressive episode after quitting. However, in those with no history of depression, major depression after quitting is rare.

If mild depression occurs, it will usually begin within the first day, continue for the first couple of weeks, and go away within a month.

What To Do

- Identify your specific feelings at the time that you seem depressed. Are you actually feeling tired, lonely, bored, or hungry? Focus on and address these specific needs.

♣ It's A Fact!!

There is some evidence that tobacco use reduces anxiety, so some of the anxiety you feel when you quit is actually what nonsmokers normally experience. Most of the anxiety you feel immediately after you quit is due to temporary changes.

> ### ✔ Quick Tip
> Everyone is different. The way that you will cope with the problems of quitting may be the opposite of what worked for your best friend or someone else. Ask your doctor about prescription medications that may help you with depression. Learn about the signs of depression and where to go for help at the National Institute of Mental Health Web site (http://www.nimh.nih.gov).

- Add up how much money you have saved already by not purchasing cigarettes and imagine (in detail) how you will spend your savings in six months.

- Call a friend and plan to have lunch, or go to a movie, a concert, or another pleasurable event.

- Make a list of things that are upsetting to you and write down solutions for them.

- Keep positive about changes in life.

- Increase physical activity. This will help to improve your mood and lift your depression.

- Focus on your strengths.

- Plan your next vacation or fun activity.

- Breathe deeply.

- Establish a list of your short- and long-term personal goals.

- Think of how healthy you will be when all smoking effects are gone from your body and you can call yourself smoke-free.

- If depression continues for more than one month, see your doctor.

Nicotine And Your Body And Mind

Nicotine is a highly addictive drug. It acts as both a stimulant and a depressant, depending upon your mood and the time of day. It controls your mood by regulating the level of activity of key parts of the brain and central nervous system that control your sense of well-being.

Facing The Morning... Without Smoking

What To Expect

Expect that your morning coffee will not taste the same without a cigarette.

Did You Know?

For many smokers, lighting up is the first event of the day. Part of many people's dependence on cigarettes evolves from a routine built mostly on making opportunities to smoke. The morning can set the tone for the rest of the day.

What To Do

- Plan a different wake-up routine.

- Take your attention off smoking right away.

- Be sure no cigarettes are available.

- Begin each day with deep breathing and one or more glasses of water.

- Make a list of early morning triggers, and avoid them.

- Begin each day with a preplanned activity that will keep you busy for an hour or more. It will keep your mind and body busy so that you don't think about smoking.

Nicotine And Your Body And Mind

After six to eight hours of sleep, your nicotine level drops and your body develops a need for a quick boost of nicotine when you wake up. Your body has become dependent on nicotine. Your mind must be ready to overcome this physical need. Before you go to sleep, make a list of things you need to avoid in the morning that will make you want to smoke. Place this list where you used to place your cigarettes.

Related Notes

Once you pinpoint high-risk situations that trigger the urge to smoke, you can start to handle such situations rationally. Waking up in the morning and starting your normal routine provides plenty of triggers to tempt you to smoke.

Facing Boredom... Without Smoking

What To Expect

You may take a break and find that you now have nothing to do. You may feel very bored when waiting for something or someone (a bus, your parents, your friends).

Did You Know?

Many smokers say they sometimes smoke to overcome boredom.

What To Do

- Plan more activities than you have time for.

- For those empty minutes, make a list of things you like to do.

- Move. Do not stay in the same place too long.

- Carry a book, magazine, or crossword puzzle for waiting times.

- Notice what is going on around you. (Look at the shape of the buildings you pass, listen to the sounds outside around you.)

- Carry something (like a cell phone) to keep your hands busy.

- Listen to a favorite song.

- Go outdoors, if you can, but not to places you associate with smoking.

Nicotine And Your Body And Mind

For smokers, boredom often brings the urge to smoke—this urge may have a physical and chemical basis. When you quit smoking, you may miss the increased excitement and good feeling that nicotine gave you. This may be true when you are feeling bored.

Related Notes

You may be very bored when taking a break. You will need to replace a smoke break with something else.

Enjoying Coffee And Tea... Without Smoking

What To Expect

- Expect that your morning coffee will not taste the same without a cigarette.

- Expect to feel a strong urge to reach for a cigarette while drinking coffee or tea.

Did You Know?

- Many smokers are used to smoking when drinking coffee or tea during or after meals, during coffee/tea breaks, or in restaurants.

- You do not have to give up coffee or tea to quit smoking.

What To Do

- If you used to smoke while drinking coffee or tea, tell people you have quit, so they won't offer you a cigarette.

- Between sips of coffee or tea, take deep breaths to inhale the aroma. Breathe deeply and slowly, while you count to five, breathe out slowly, counting to five again.

- Try switching to decaffeinated coffee for a while, particularly if quitting has made you irritable or nervous.

- Try nibbling on healthy foods to keep your hands busy while you drink coffee or tea.

- As you drink your coffee, get out a scratch pad, doodle, or make plans for the day.

- If the urge to smoke is very strong, drink your coffee or tea faster than usual and then change activities or rooms.

Nicotine And Your Body And Mind

Many studies have reported that smoking may make you feel happier and more alert. Smokers may associate these good feelings with drinking coffee or tea. When you quit smoking, you may feel saddened by the loss of these good feelings, and drinking coffee or tea without smoking may make you feel even sadder. Try not to feel sad; think of what you've gained by quitting.

Enjoying Meals.... Without Smoking

What To Expect

Smoking urges may be stronger at different meal times—sometimes breakfast, sometimes lunch, or sometimes dinner. Your smoking urges may be stronger with certain foods, such as spicy or sweet meals or snacks.

- Expect to want to smoke after meals or with others at a restaurant.

- Expect the urge to smoke when you smell cigarette smoke at a restaurant.

- When you no longer smoke at the table after meals, you can expect that others will be pleased.

Did You Know?

Many smokers feel the need to smoke after meals at home, work, or a restaurant. Your desire to smoke after meals may depend on whether you are alone, with other smokers, or with nonsmokers.

What To Do

- Know what kinds of foods increase your urge to smoke and stay away from them.

- If you are alone, call a friend or take a walk as soon as you've finished eating.

- Brush your teeth or use mouthwash right after meals.

✔ Quick Tip

Talk to your doctor about nicotine replacement therapy and other medications to help you quit smoking. Nicotine cravings may be reduced by using nicotine replacement products, which deliver small, steady doses of nicotine into the body. Nicotine replacement patches, gum, lozenges, nasal spray, and inhaler appear to be equally effective. Bupropion pills (which don't contain nicotine) also help relieve withdrawal symptoms.

- If possible, have someone massage your shoulders.

- If you have coffee or a fruit drink, concentrate on the taste.

- Wash the dishes by hand after eating—you can't smoke with wet hands!

Nicotine And Your Body And Mind

Nicotine stops hunger pains in your stomach for as long as one hour, and it also makes your blood sugar level go up. When you quit, this is reversed. Smoking and eating are both ways to meet certain needs (stimulation, relaxation, pampering, time out, comfort, or socialization), so when you quit smoking, you may eat more. Withdrawal from nicotine enhances the taste of sweeter foods. Food often tastes better after you quit smoking, and you may have a bigger appetite.

Related Notes

Once you pinpoint high-risk situations that trigger the urge to smoke, you can begin to handle such situations. Eating and drinking are often very important triggers. Nicotine replacement products may be used to help you handle cravings.

Driving Or Riding In A Car... Without Smoking

What To Expect

Expect to want to reach for a cigarette when driving a car or traveling as a passenger. On longer trips, you may find yourself getting more sleepy than usual.

Did You Know?

Like many smokers, you may like to light up when driving as a means to relieve stress, stay alert, relax, or just pass the time. Your desire to smoke may be stronger and more frequent on longer trips.

What To Do

- Remove the ashtray, lighter, and cigarettes from your car.

- Turn your radio on or put on your favorite tape or CD and sing along.

- Clean your car and make sure to use deodorizers to reduce the tobacco smell.

- Tell yourself:
    - "This urge will go away in a few minutes."
    - "So, I'm not enjoying this car ride. Big deal! It won't last forever!"
    - "My car smells clean and fresh!"
    - "I'm a better driver now that I'm not smoking while driving."
- Ask friends and passengers not to smoke in your car.
- If you're not driving, find something to do with your hands.
- Take an alternate route to work.
- Try carpooling.
- For a little while, avoid taking long car trips. If you do, take plenty of rest stops.
- Keep non-fattening snacks in your car (sunflower seeds, licorice, and sugarless gum and hard candy).
- Take fresh fruit with you on long trips.
- Plan stops for water or fruit juice.

Nicotine And Your Body And Mind

You may have become used to smoking while driving—to relax in a traffic jam or to stay alert on a long drive. There is some evidence that smoking actually does make you feel more awake and alert. In the past, you may have relied upon this during both short and long rides. Remember, on longer trips, you may not be able to stay awake for as long as you used to.

Being Around Other Smokers... Without Smoking

What To Expect

Some friends, especially those who are smokers themselves, may not be supportive of your efforts to cut down or quit. Also, they may not understand how much impact their behavior can have on your efforts to quit.

Did You Know?

You may find that you don't want to smoke just because you see someone else smoking. Rather, your desire to smoke may be triggered by something special about the situation. For example, being around the people you usually smoked with could trigger the urge to smoke.

What To Do

- Ask others to help you in your quit attempt. Give them specific examples of things that are helpful (such as not smoking around you) and things that are not helpful (like asking you to buy cigarettes for them).

- Post a small "No Smoking" sign by your door. Provide an outside area where smokers may go if they wish to smoke.

- If you are in a group and others light up, excuse yourself, and don't return until they have finished.

- Do not buy, carry, light, or hold cigarettes for others.

- Try not to get angry if family, friends, or coworkers hassle you about quitting.

Nicotine And Your Body And Mind

You may want to analyze situations in which watching others smoke triggers your urge to smoke. Figure out what it is about that situation that makes you want to smoke. Many studies have reported that smoking may make you feel happier, more alert, and not as anxious. These good feelings may make you want to smoke. Also, you may associate these feelings with being around other smokers. When you quit, you may feel saddened by the loss of these good feelings; being around smokers may make you feel even sadder. Try not to feel sad; think of what you've gained by quitting.

Related Notes

Once you pinpoint high-risk "trigger" situations, you can start to handle them rationally. Nicotine cravings may be reduced by using nicotine replacement products, which deliver small, steady doses of nicotine into the body.

☞ Remember!!

The changes you intend to make may disturb friends and family members who are smokers. Friends may feel that your efforts to quit smoking will put a strain on your friendship. It will be tempting to join others for routine smoke breaks.

Chapter 53

Spit Tobacco: A Guide For Quitting

So you're a dipper and you'd like to quit. Maybe you've already found that quitting dip or chew is not easy. But you can do it! This information is intended to help you make your own plan for quitting.

Many former dippers have shared advice on quitting that can help you. This chapter is the result of advice from chewers and dippers who have canned the habit.

Like most dippers, you probably know that the health-related reasons to quit are awesome. But you must find your own personal reasons for quitting. They can motivate you more than the fear of health consequences. It's important to develop your own recipe for willpower.

In this chapter we refer more to dip than chew, just to keep it simple. Also, note that we call it spit tobacco, not smokeless tobacco. Smokeless tobacco is the term preferred by the tobacco industry. It makes the products sound safe. They aren't.

The Dangers Of Dip And Chew

Here's a brief summary of the harm dipping does in the mouth.

- Spit tobacco use may cause cancer of the mouth.
- Sugar in spit tobacco may cause decay in exposed tooth roots.

About This Chapter: From "Spit Tobacco: A Guide for Quitting," National Institute of Dental and Craniofacial Research (www.nidcr.nih.gov), June 18, 2009.

- Dip and chew can cause your gums to pull away from the teeth in the place where the tobacco is held. The gums do not grow back.

- Leathery white patches and red sores are common in dippers and chewers and can turn into cancer.

Spit Tobacco Use Can Cause Problems In Other Parts Of The Body

Recent research shows that spit tobacco use might also cause problems beyond the mouth. Some studies have shown that using spit tobacco may cause pancreatic cancer. And scientists are also looking at the possibility that spit tobacco use might play a role in the development of cardiovascular disease (heart disease) and stroke.

Need More Reasons To Quit?

It's Expensive

A can of dip costs an average of nearly $3. A two-can-a-week habit costs about $300 per year. A can-a-day habit costs nearly $1,100 per year. Likewise, chewing tobacco costs about $2. A pouch-a-day habit costs over $700 a year. Think of all the things you could do with that money instead of dipping or chewing. It adds up.

It's Disgusting

If the health effects don't worry you, think of how other people see your addiction. The smell of spit tobacco in your mouth is not pleasant. While you may have become used to the odor and don't mind it, others around you notice.

Check out your clothes. Do you have tobacco juice stains on your clothes, your furniture, or on your car's upholstery? Your tobacco spit and drool could be making a mess.

Look at your teeth. Are they stained from tobacco juice? Brushing your teeth won't make this go away.

Understanding Your Addiction

Nicotine, found in all tobacco products, is a highly addictive drug that acts in the brain and throughout the body.

How Addicted Are You?

Dip and chew contain more nicotine than cigarettes.

• Do you longer get sick or dizzy when you dip or chew, like you did when you first started.

• Do you dip more often and in different settings.

• Have you switched to stronger products, with more nicotine.

• Do you swallow juice from my tobacco on a regular basis.

• Do you sometimes sleep with dip or chew in my mouth.

• Do you take your first dip or chew first thing in the morning.

• Do you find it hard to go more than a few hours without dip or chew.

• Do you have strong cravings when you go without dip or chew.
The more items that apply, the more likely that you are addicted.

Myths And Truths

There are several myths about spit tobacco. Sometimes these myths make users feel more comfortable in their habits. Below are some myths and the truths that relate to them.

• **Myth:** Spit tobacco is a harmless alternative to smoking.

• **Truth:** Spit tobacco is still tobacco. In tobacco are nitrosamines, cancer-causing chemicals from the curing process. Note the warnings on the cans.

• **Myth:** Dip (or chew) improves my athletic performance.

• **Truth:** A study of professional baseball players found no connection between spit tobacco use and player performance. Using spit tobacco

---

❖ It's A Fact!!

Holding an average-size dip in your mouth for 30 minutes gives you as much nicotine as smoking three cigarettes. A two-can-a-week snuff dipper gets as much nicotine as a one and a half pack-a-day smoker does.

increases your heart rate and blood pressure within a few minutes. This can cause a buzz or rush, but the rise in pulse and blood pressure places an extra stress on your heart.

- **Myth:** Good gum care can offset the harmful effects of using dip or chew.
- **Truth:** There is no evidence that brushing and flossing will undo the harm that dip and chew are doing to your teeth and gums.
- **Myth:** It's easy to quit using dip or chew when you want to.
- **Truth:** Unfortunately, nicotine addiction makes quitting difficult. But those who have quit successfully are very glad they did.

Quitting Plan

Kicking the spit or chew habit can be tough, but it can be done, and you can do it. The best way to quit spit tobacco is to have a quit date and a quitting plan. These methods make it easier. Try what you think will work best for you.

Decide To Quit

Quitting spit tobacco is not something you do on a whim. You have to want to quit to make it through those first few weeks off tobacco. You know your reasons for stopping. Don't let outside influence, like peer-pressure, get in your way. Focus on all you don't like about dipping and chewing.

Reasons To Quit

Here are some reasons given by others. Are any of them important to you?

- To avoid health problems
- To prove I can do it
- I have sores or white patches in my mouth
- To please someone I care about
- To set a good example for other kids
- To save money
- I don't like the taste

- I have gum or tooth problems

- It's disgusting

- Because it's banned at work or school

- I don't want it to control me

- My girlfriend (or a girl I'd like to date) hates it

- My physician or dentist told me to quit

Pick A Quit Date

Pick your quit date. Even if you think you're ready to quit now, take at least a week to get ready. But don't put off setting a date.

Get Psyched Up For Quitting

Cut back before you quit by tapering down. Have your physician or dentist check your mouth. Ask whether you need nicotine replacement therapy (gum, nicotine patches). There is no "ideal" time to quit, but low-stress times are best. Having a quit date in mind is important, no matter how far off it is. But it's best to pick a date in the next two weeks, so you don't put it off too long.

Cut Back Before You Quit

Some people are able to quit spit tobacco "cold turkey." Others find that cutting back makes quitting easier. There are many ways to cut back.

Taper down. Cut back to half of your usual amount before you quit. If you usually carry your tin or pouch with you, try leaving it behind. Carry substitutes instead—sugar-free chewing gum or hard candies, and sunflower seeds. During this period, you might also try a mint-leaf snuff.

Cut back on when and where you dip or chew. First, notice when your cravings are strongest. What events trigger dipping or chewing for you? Do you always reach for a dip after meals? When you work out? In your car or truck? On your job? Don't carry your pouch or tin. Use a substitute instead. Go as long as you possibly can without giving into a craving—at least ten minutes. Try to go longer and longer as you approach your quit day. Now, pick three of your strongest triggers and stop dipping or chewing at those times. This will be hard at first. The day will come when you are used to going without tobacco at the times you want it most.

Notice what friends and co-workers who don't dip or chew are doing at these times. This will give you ideas for dip or chew substitutes. It's a good idea to avoid your dipping and chewing pals while you're trying to quit. That will help you avoid the urge to reach for a can or chew.

Switch to a lower nicotine tobacco product. This way, you cut down your nicotine dose while you're getting ready to quit. This can help to prevent strong withdrawal when you quit.

Don't switch to other tobacco products like cigarettes or cigars! In fact, if you already smoke, this is a good time to quit smoking. That way you can get over all your nicotine addiction at once.

Build A Support Team

Let friends, family, and co-workers know you're quitting. Warn them that you may not be your usual self for a week or two after you quit. Ask them to be patient. Ask them to stand by to listen and encourage you when the going gets rough.

Suggest ways they can help, like joining you for a run or a walk, helping you find ways to keep busy, and telling you they know you can do it. If they've quit, ask them for tips. If they use dip or chew, ask them not to offer you any. They don't have to quit themselves to be supportive, but maybe someone will want to quit with you.

Quit Day

Make your quit day special right from the beginning. You're doing yourself a huge favor. Change daily routines to break away from tobacco triggers. When you eat breakfast, don't sit in the usual place at the kitchen table. Get right up from the table after meals.

Make an appointment to get your teeth cleaned. You'll enjoy the fresh, clean feeling and a whiter smile.

Keep busy and active. Start the day with a walk, run, swim, or workout. Aerobic exercise will help you relax. Plus, it boosts energy, stamina, and all-around fitness and curbs your appetite.

Chew substitutes. Try sugar-free hard candies or gum, cinnamon sticks, mints, beef jerky, or sunflower seeds. Carry them with you and use them whenever you have the urge to dip or chew.

What About Medications?

Nicotine replacement therapy and non-nicotine replacement therapy (bupropion) are approved by the U.S. Food and Drug Administration (FDA) for smoking cessation. However, these products have not been approved for spit tobacco cessation. Further research is needed to determine their effectiveness for helping spit tobacco users quit.

Your First Week Off Spit Tobacco: Coping With Withdrawal

Withdrawal symptoms don't last long: Symptoms are strongest the first week after you quit. The worst part is over after two weeks. As time passes, you'll feel better than when you dipped or chewed. So be patient with yourself.

Urges to dip, cravings—especially in the places you used to dip the most: Wait it out. Deep breathing and exercise help you feel better right away.

Feeling irritable, tense, restless, impatient: Walk away from the situation. Deep breathing and exercise help to blow off steam. Ask others to be patient.

Constipation and irregularity: Add fiber to your diet (whole grain breads and cereals, fresh fruits and vegetables).

Hunger and weight gain: Eat regular meals. Feeling hungry is sometimes mistaken for the desire to dip or chew.

Desire for sweets: Reach for low-calorie sweet snacks (like apples, sugar-free gums and candies).

Your Second Week: Dealing With Triggers

You've made it through the hardest part: the first week. If you can stay off one week, then you can stay off two. Just use the same willpower and strategies that got you this far. Cravings may be just as strong this week, but they will come less often and go away sooner.

☞ Remember!!

Nicotine speeds up metabolism, so quitting spit tobacco may result in a slight weight gain. To limit the amount of weight you gain, try the following:

- Eat well-balanced meals and avoid fatty foods.

- To satisfy your cravings for sweets, eat small pieces of fruit.

- Keep low-calorie foods handy for snacks.

- Try popcorn (without butter), sugar-free gums and mints, fresh fruits, and vegetables.

- Drink six to eight glasses of water each day.

- Work about 30 minutes of daily exercise into your routine; try walking or another activity such as running, cycling, or swimming.

Be Prepared For Temptation

Tobacco thoughts and urges probably still bother you. They will be strongest in the places where you dipped or chewed the most. The more time you spend in these places without dipping or chewing, the weaker the urges will become. Avoid alcoholic beverages. Drinking them could bust your plan to quit. Know what events and places will be triggers for you and plan ahead for them.

Write down some of your triggers. And write what you'll do instead of dip or chew. It may be as simple as reaching for gum or seeds, walking away, or thinking about how far you've come.

Tips For Going The Distance

Congratulations. You've broken free of a tough addiction. If you can stay off two weeks, then you know you can beat this addiction. It will get easier. Keep using whatever worked when you first quit. Don't expect new rituals to take the place of spit tobacco right away. It took time to get used to chewing or dipping at first, too.

Keep up your guard. Continue to plan ahead for situations that may tempt you.

What If You Should Slip?

Try not to slip, not even once. But, if you do slip, get right back on track. Don't let feelings of guilt lead you back to chewing or dipping. A slip does not mean "failure." Figure out why you slipped and how to avoid it next time. Get rid of any leftover tobacco.

Celebrate Your Success

Congratulations. You've done it. You've beaten the spit tobacco habit. You're improving your health and your future. Celebrate with the people on your "support team." Offer your support to friends and co-workers who are trying to quit using tobacco. Pledge to yourself never to take another dip or chew.

☞ **Remember!!**

Pick up right where you left off before the slip. If slips are frequent, or you are dipping or chewing on a regular basis, make a new quitting plan. Quitting takes practice. The spit tobacco habit can be tough to beat. Most users don't quit for good on the first try. Don't give up. Figure out what would have helped. Try a new approach next time. Talk to your physician or dentist for extra help.

Chapter 54

How To Encourage Someone Who Is Trying To Quit Smoking

Help Someone Quit: Make A Difference

When someone you care about has made the decision to stop smoking or chewing tobacco, your support of their decision plays an enormous role in their success. This chapter will help you understand your role as they progress through the four steps to quit and prepare you to be the best cheerleader, quit partner, or safety net you can be.

Step 1: Thinking About Quitting

- When it comes to quitting, it needs to be their decision, so be sure to support rather than pressure them.

- Choose the right times to encourage them, such as when they talk about "how they should quit" or are sick and "need to stop smoking."

- Don't give up or get frustrated if they fail to follow through when they had talked about quitting. Give them some time and start the discussion again when the opportunity arises.

About This Chapter: This chapter begins with "How to Help Someone Quit," produced by the U.S. Department of Defense's *Quit Tobacco—Make Everyone Proud* program, July 2009. Additional information from the Nemours Foundation is cited separately within the chapter.

Step 2: Preparing To Quit

- If you use tobacco, please consider quitting along with them. As quit buddies, you can motivate one another like exercise workout partners.

- Help them pick a quit date that's right for them and stick to it.

- If the opportunity presents itself, suggest medications and professional support to aide them in the quitting process. Do your research. Know what to expect along the way and learn about specific strategies to fight the nicotine withdrawal cravings in tough times.

- Help them remove all tobacco-related products from their home and car, such as lighters, ashtrays, and empty tobacco packages.

- Encourage them to let their friends and co-workers know they are quitting as well.

Step 3: Quitting

- Compliment them often on their efforts to quit. Positive feedback is always welcome and appreciated. Help them develop a reward system right away. Rewards aren't just for long milestones; they're for making it past everyday obstacles as well.

- If you use tobacco products, be sure to help your quitter by not using in front of him or her or leaving cigarettes and chew in plain sight.

- Avoid taking them places where they would normally be encouraged to smoke.

- Be prepared to help your quitter find healthy distractions when he or she experiences tobacco cravings. Have a healthy snack, play a game, crack them up with a new joke or suggest that they start a quit journal to monitor and record their progress.

- Spend time having fun with your quitter. Physical activities, such as sports or even a walk, will make you both feel better. It helps relieve the stress of nicotine withdrawal.

- Let them know that you're available for them when they need an encouraging word or a strong shoulder. If you're not available, let them know they can always get support from cessation coaches available via live chat on the site www.ucanquit2.org (also, see the last chapter of this book for additional suggestions).

- Show them you still care and support them even if they are moody or agitated.

- Spend more time with friends who know they're quitting and are supporting them. It's no fun trying to quit smoking when their buddies are waving cigarettes under their nose and trying to get them to slip up.

- Be understanding. Setbacks are not failures. They are just part of the process of changing behavior.

Step 4: Staying Quit

- Celebrate their success with them when they have quit smoking or chewing tobacco, especially at tobacco-free milestones.

- For most people, quitting takes much more than one try. Often it can take five to 10 quitting attempts to stay quit, so be ready to offer nonjudgmental encouragement and assurance that slip-ups and relapses are normal.

- If your quitter has a relapse, you can reinforce the positives of trying to quit.

- If your quitter has started smoking or chewing again, help them, set a new quit date and try again. Suggest alternative treatments or use the opportunity to reinforce that additional professional help and medications that could make an impact.

Helping A Parent Who Smokes

Text under this heading is from "Helping a Parent Who Smokes" November 2007, reprinted with permission from www.kidshealth.org. Copyright © 2007 The Nemours Foundation. This information was provided by KidsHealth, one of the largest resources online for medically reviewed health information written for parents, kids, and teens. For more articles like this one, visit www.KidsHealth.org, or www.TeensHealth.org.

You can't escape the message that smoking is bad for you. But what if one or both of your parents smoke? You might be worried about their health, sick of smelling the smoke, or even a little embarrassed by it. You can't order your mom or dad to stop smoking, but you can encourage them to quit. There are lots of good reasons. Here are some you can mention:

- Smoking will hurt their health.

- Smoking creates secondhand smoke, which you don't like.

- Smoking will make it hard for them to keep up with you because they might run out of breath easily.

If you think it will help, you could print out articles like this one to give it to your mom or dad. Many states now have free programs to help people quit smoking. You might see them advertised on billboards in your town.

✔ Quick Tip

Quit Tobacco With A Buddy

Have you heard that old song "One Is the Loneliest Number"? Maybe they wrote that song about quitting tobacco! It's hard to do, and even harder if you go it alone. Find a friend who wants to quit smoking or chewing tobacco too and you've instantly improved your chances for success. You'll both be working toward the same goal—staying tobacco free! Of course you can quit smoking or chewing tobacco alone, but it just makes sense to work as a team. The buddy system is custom made for quitting tobacco.

You and your quit buddy should start by making a quit list of all of the good reasons to quit. You can count on one another to stay focused and strong. The two of you might have different strategies or reasons for quitting, but you're still on the same team with the same goal. If he wants to quit cold turkey and you want to use medicine to help quit smoking, that's fine.

Fill out your quit plans together and identify things that are most likely to make you crave a smoke, dip, or chew. Once you've spelled out your triggers, you can warn your quit buddy that you'll need the most help during those times. Plan to meet in person and talk on the phone regularly. After all, nobody knows what you're going through better than your quit buddy.

Source: From "Quit Tobacco with a Buddy," produced by the U.S. Department of Defense's *Quit Tobacco—Make Everyone Proud* program, August 12, 2009.

Point these out to your parents and encourage them to find out more about these programs.

But what if your parent gets angry with you for bringing up the topic of smoking? People don't like to be reminded that they are doing something unhealthy, so it's possible your parents will be insulted or angry, especially if they're worried they won't be able to quit. Maybe they have tried before and failed.

Remember to be kind and respectful when you discuss smoking with your mom or dad. Also remember that it is difficult to quit. Some people try several times before they're able to quit for good. Instead of yelling at them, tell them that you love them and want them to enjoy many healthy years ahead. In time, your mom or dad may realize you are right about smoking.

And if they do agree to stop smoking, be their biggest supporter. Ask if there's anything you can do to help them when they feel the urge to smoke. Maybe you could go for a walk, do a puzzle, or listen to music together. As they reach milestones, such as a month without smoking, be sure to celebrate the achievement. Way to go, mom! Way to go, dad!

Part Six

If You Need More Help Or Information

Chapter 55

The Health Effects Of Tobacco Use: A Directory Of Resources

National and International Organizations

Action on Smoking and Health
2013 H Street, NW
Washington, DC 20006
Phone: 202-659-4310
Website: http://ash.org
Website: www.no-smoking.org

Advocacy Institute
1629 K St., NW, Suite 200
Washington, DC 20006-1629
Phone: 202-777-7575
Website: www.advocacy.org/
tobacco.htm
E-mail: info@advocacy.org

American Academy of Family Physicians
11400 Tomahawk Creek Parkway
Leawood, KS 66211-2672
Website: www.aafp.org

American Cancer Society
250 Williams St., NW
Atlanta, GA 30303
Toll-Free: 800-227-2345
(800-ACS-2345)
Website: www.cancer.org

American College of Chest Physicians
3300 Dundee Road
Northbrook, IL 60062-2348
Phone: 847-498-1400
Website: www.chestnet.org

American Council on Science and Health
1995 Broadway, 2nd Floor
New York, NY 10023-5860
Phone: 212-362-7044
Website: www.acsh.org

American Dental Hygienists' Association
444 North Michigan Avenue,
Suite 3400
Chicago, IL 60611
Website: www.adha.org

American Heart Association National Center
7272 Greenville Avenue
Dallas, TX 75231
Toll-Free: 800-AHA-USA1
Website: www.americanheart.org

American Legacy Foundation
1724 Massachusetts Ave., NW
Washington, DC 20036
Phone: 202-454-5555
Website: www.legacyforhealth.org

American Lung Association (ALA)
1301 Pennsylvania Ave., NW
Washington, DC 20004
Toll-Free: 800-LUNG-USA
Phone: 202-785-3355
Website: www.lungusa.org

American Public Health Association
800 I Street, NW
Washington, DC 20001-3710
Phone: 202-777-APHA
Website: www.apha.org

Americans for Nonsmokers' Rights
2530 San Pablo Avenue, Suite J
Berkeley, CA 94702
Phone: 510-841-3032
Website: www.no-smoke.org

Australian Tobacco Control Supersite
School of Public Health
Edward Ford Building A27
The University of Sydney
NSW 2006
Australia
Phone: (+61 2) 9351 5203
Website: www.health.usyd.edu.au/tobacco

BADvertising Institute
Website: www.badvertising.org

Campaign for Tobacco-Free Kids
1400 Eye Street
Suite 1200
Washington DC 20005
Phone: 202-296-5469
Website: www.tobaccofreekids.org

Canadian Council for Tobacco Control
192 Bank Street
Ottawa, Ontario
Canada K2P 1W8
Toll-Free: 800-267-5234
Phone: (613) 567-3050
Website: www.cctc.ca
E-mail: infoservices@cctc.ca

Canadian Lung Association
1750 Courtwood Crescent
Suite 300
Ottawa, ON
K2C 2B5
Canada
Phone: 613-569-6411
Website: www.lung.ca
E-mail: info@lung.ca

Cancer Council New South Wales
P.O. Box 572
Kings Cross, New South Wales, 1340
Australia
Phone: (+61 2) 9334 1900
Website: www.cancercouncil.com.au

Cancer Research UK
P.O. Box 123
Lincoln's Inn Fields
London WC2A 3PX
Phone: 020 7242 0200 (UK)
Website: http://info.cancer
researchuk.org

Center for Tobacco Research and Intervention
University of Wisconsin Medical
School
1930 Monroe St.
Madison, WI 53711
Phone: 608-262-8673
Website: http://www.ctri.wisc.edu

European Network for Smoking Prevention
Chaussee d'Ixelles 144
1050 Brussels
Belgium
Phone: (32) 2/230.65.15
Website: www.ensp.org
E-mail: info@ensp.org

Group Against Smokers' Pollution (GASP)
5604 Solway St. #204
Pittsburgh, PA 15217
Phone: 412-325-7382
Website: www.gasp-pgh.org
E-mail: gasp@gasp-pgh.org

International Network of Women Against Tobacco

c/o British Columbia Centre for
Excellence in Women's Health
E-311 4500 Oak Street, Box 48
Vancouver, BC V6H 3N1
Canada
Phone: 604-875-2633
Website: www.inwat.org

Robert Wood Johnson Foundation

P.O. Box 2316
College Road East and Route 1
Princeton, NJ 08543-2316
Website: www.rwjf.org

Join Together

Boston University
580 Harrison Avenue, 3rd Floor
Boston, MA 02118
Phone: 617-437-1500
Website: www.jointogether.org

National Cancer Institute

NCI Office of Communications
and Education
Public Inquiries Office
6116 Executive Boulevard
Suite 300
Bethesda, MD 20892-8322
Toll-Free: 800-4-CANCER
TTY: 800-332-8615
Smoking Quitline:
877-44U-QUIT
Website: www.cancer.gov

National Center for Chronic Disease Prevention and Health Promotion

1600 Clifton Rd.
Atlanta, GA 30333
Toll-Free: 800-CDC-INFO
(800-232-4636)
Website: www.cdc.gov/tobacco

National Families in Action

P.O. Box 133136
Atlanta, GA 30333
Phone: 404-248-9676
Website: www.nationalfamilies.org
E-mail: nfia@nationalfamilies.org

National Heart, Lung, and Blood Institute

P.O. Box 30105
Bethesda, MD 20824-0105
Phone: 301-592-8573
TTY: 240-629-3255
Website: www.nhlbi.nih.gov

National Institute of Dental and Craniofacial Research

Toll-Free: 866-232-4528
Website: www.nidcr.nih.gov
E-mail: nidcrinfo@mail.nih.gov

National Institute of Mental Health

6001 Executive Boulevard
Room 8184, MSC 9663
Bethesda, MD 20892-9663
Toll-Free: 866-615-6464
Toll-Free TTY: 866-415-8051
Phone: 301-443-4513
TTY: 301-443-8431
Website: www.nimh.nih.gov
E-mail: nimhinfo@nih.gov

National Institute on Drug Abuse

6001 Executive Blvd., Room 5213
Bethesda, MD 20892-9561
Phone: 301-443-1124
Website: www.nida.nih.gov

National Spit Tobacco Education Program

Oral Health America
410 North Michigan Avenue
Suite 352
Chicago, IL 60611
Phone: 312-836-9900

Office of the Surgeon General

5600 Fishers Lane, Room 18-66
Rockville, MD 20857
Phone: 301-443-4000
Website: www.surgeongeneral.gov

Ohio State University Medical Center

410 W. 10th Ave.
Columbus, OH 43210
Toll-Free: 800-293-5123
Library for Health Information:
614-293-3707
Website: http://medicalcenter.osu.edu
E-mail: health-info@osu.edu

Smoke-Free Environments Law Project

Center for Social Gerontology
2307 Shelby Avenue
Ann Arbor, MI 48103
Phone: 734-665-1126
Website: www.tcsg.org/sfelp/home
.htm
E-mail: SFELP@tcsg.org

Society for Research on Nicotine and Tobacco

2424 American Lane
Madison, WI 53704
Phone: 608-443-2462
Website: www.srnt.org
E-mail: info@srnt.org

Substance Abuse and Mental Health Services Administration

P.O. Box 2345
Rockville, MD 20847-2345
Phone: 877-SMHSA-7 (726-4727)
Website: www.samhsa.gov

Tobacco Control Legal Consortium

875 Summit Ave.
St. Paul, MN 55105
Phone: 651-290-7506
Website: www.tobaccolawcenter.org
Website: www.tclconline.org

Tobacco Control Resource Center

Northeastern University
360 Huntington Ave.
117 Cushing Hall
Boston, MA 02115
Phone: 617-373-2026
Website: www.tobaccocontrol.neu
.edu

Tobacco Control Resource Center for Wisconsin

333 East Campus Mall, #8104
Madison, WI 53715-1381
Toll-Free: 800-248-9244
Website: www.tobwis.org
E-mail: tcrcw@tobwis.org

Tobacco Etiology Research Network

University of Kentucky
Center for Prevention Research
121 Washington Avenue,
Suite 204
Lexington, KY 40536-0003
Website: www.tern.org

Tobacco Technical Assistance Consortium

Emory University
MS: 1599-001-1BW
1599 Clifton Road, 6th Floor
Atlanta, GA 30322
Phone: 404-712-8474
Website: www.ttac.org
E-mail: ttac@sph.emory.edu

U.S. Environmental Protection Agency

Ariel Rios Building
1200 Pennsylvania Avenue, NW
Washington, DC 20460
Toll-Free: 800-438-4318
Phone: 202-343-9370
Website: www.epa.gov

Online Resources

Dog Breath
Website: www.dogbreath.org

Go Ask Alice
Columbia University Health Education Program
Website: www.goaskalice.columbia.edu

Joe Chemo
Website: www.joechemo.org

KidsHealth/Nemours Foundation
Website: www.kidshealth.org

Nicotine and the Brain
Neuroscience for Kids, Washington University
Website: http://faculty.washington.edu/chudler/nic.html

Scoop on Smoking
American Council on Science and Health
Website: Health Effects Gateway Page: www.thescooponsmoking.org/
xhtml/effectsHome.php

Tobacco-Free Kids
Website: www.tobaccofreekids.org

Tobacco Free U
Website: www.tobaccofreeu.org

Tobacco News and Information
Website: www.tobacco.org

Truth
Website: www.thetruth.com

World Health Organization, Tobacco Free Initiative
Website: www.who.int/tobacco/en

Chapter 56

Smoking Cessation Resources

Cessation Help By Phone

American Cancer Society
Toll-Free: 800-ACS-2345

American Heart Association & American Stroke Association
Toll-Free: 800-AHA-USA-1
(800-242-8721)

American Lung Association
Toll-Free: 800-LUNG-USA

National Network of Tobacco Cessation Quitlines
Toll-Free: 800-QUITNOW
(800-784-8669)

New York State Smokers' Quitline
Toll-Free: 866-NY-QUITS
(866-697-8487)

Nicotine Anonymous
Toll-Free: 877-TRY-NICA
(877-879-6422)

Smoking Quitline
Toll-Free: 877-44U-QUIT
Monday through Friday, 9:00 a.m. to 4:30 p.m. Eastern Time

Online Resources

Center for Tobacco Cessation
Website: www.ctcinfo.org

Clear Horizons
University of Rochester
Website: www.myclearhorizons
.com

Coalition for Tobacco-Free Arizona
Website: www.tobaccofreeaz.org

Committed Quitters
Website: www.quit.com

Help for Smokers and Other Tobacco Users
Website: www.ahrq.gov/consumer/
tobacco/helpsmokers.htm

Helping Young Smokers Quit
Website: www.
helpingyoungsmokersquit.org

How Bob Quit Smoking
Website: www.bobquits.com

Kick Butts Day
Website: www.kickbuttsday.org

My Last Dip
Website: www.mylastdip.com

✔ **Quick Tip**

For counseling and information about resources for smoking cessation within your state, call 800-QUITNOW.

National Lung Health Education Program
Website: www.nlhep.org

Nicotine Anonymous
Website: www.nicotine-anonymous
.org

Partnership for a Drug-Free America
Website: www.drugfreeamerica.org

Quit Tobacco. Make Everyone Proud
Website: www.ucanquit2.org

QuitNet
Website: www.quitnet.com

Quitting Tobacco: Challenges, Strategies, and Benefits
Website: www.cme.nci.nih.gov/
cancertopics/tobacco/quittingtips

qWeb.org
Website: www.qweb.org

Smoke-Free Families
Website: www.smokefreefamilies.org

Smokefree
Website: www.smokefree.gov

Smokefree Women
Website: women.smokefree.gov

Tobacco Free Earth
Website: www.tobaccofreeearth.com

Tri-County Cessation Center
Website: www.tricountycessation.org

Why Quit
Website: www.whyquit.com

Youth Quit 4 Life
Website: www.quit4life.com

Youth Tobacco Cessation: A Guide for Making Informed Decisions
Website: www.cdc.gov/tobacco/
quit_smoking/cessation/youth_
tobacco_cessation/index.htm

Youth Tobacco Cessation Collaborative
Website: www.
youthtobaccocessation.org

Index

Index

Page numbers that appear in *Italics* refer to tables or illustrations. Page numbers that have a small 'n' after the page number refer to information shown as Notes at the beginning of each chapter. Page numbers that appear in **Bold** refer to information contained in boxes on that page (except Notes information at the beginning of each chapter).

F

G

H